twenty

January

MON	TUE	WED	THU	FRI	SAT	SUN
				1	2	3
4	5	6	7	8	9	10
11	12	13	14	15	16	17
18	19	20	21	22	23	24
25	26	27	28	29	30	31

February

MON	TUE	WED	THU	FRI	SAT	SUN
1	2	3	4	5	6	7
8	9	10	11	12	13	14
15	16	17	18	19	20	21
22	23	24	25	26	27	28

March

MON	TUE	WED	THU	FRI	SAT	SUN
1	2	3	4	5	6	7
8	9	10	11	12	13	14
15	16	17	18	19	20	21
22	23	24	25	26	27	28
29	30	31				

April

MON	TUE	WED	THU	FRI	SAT	SUN
			1	2	3	4
5	6	7	8	9	10	11
12	13	14	15	16	17	18
19	20	21	22	23	24	25
26	27	28	29	30		

May

MON	TUE	WED	THU	FRI	SAT	SUN
					1	2
3	4	5	6	7	8	9
10	11	12	13	14	15	16
17	18	19	20	21	22	23
24/31	25	26	27	28	29	30

June

MON	TUE	WED	THU	FRI	SAT	SUN
	1	2	3	4	5	6
7	8	9	10	11	12	13
14	15	16	17	18	19	20
21	22	23	24	25	26	27
28	29	30				

July

MON	TUE	WED	THU	FRI	SAT	SUN
			1	2	3	4
5	6	7	8	9	10	11
12	13	14	15	16	17	18
19	20	21	22	23	24	25
26	27	28	29	30	31	

August

MON	TUE	WED	THU	FRI	SAT	SUN
						1
2	3	4	5	6	7	8
9	10	11	12	13	14	15
16	17	18	19	20	21	22
23/30	24/31	25	26	27	28	29

September

MON	TUE	WED	THU	FRI	SAT	SUN
		1	2	3	4	5
6	7	8	9	10	11	12
13	14	15	16	17	18	19
20	21	22	23	24	25	26
27	28	29	30			

October

MON	TUE	WED	THU	FRI	SAT	SUN
				1	2	3
4	5	6	7	8	9	10
11	12	13	14	15	16	17
18	19	20	21	22	23	24
25	26	27	28	29	30	31

November

MON	TUE	WED	THU	FRI	SAT	SUN
1	2	3	4	5	6	7
8	9	10	11	12	13	14
15	16	17	18	19	20	21
22	23	24	25	26	27	28
29	30					

December

MON	TUE	WED	THU	FRI	SAT	SUN
		1	2	3	4	5
6	7	8	9	10	11	12
13	14	15	16	17	18	19
20	21	22	23	24	25	26
27	28	29	30	31		

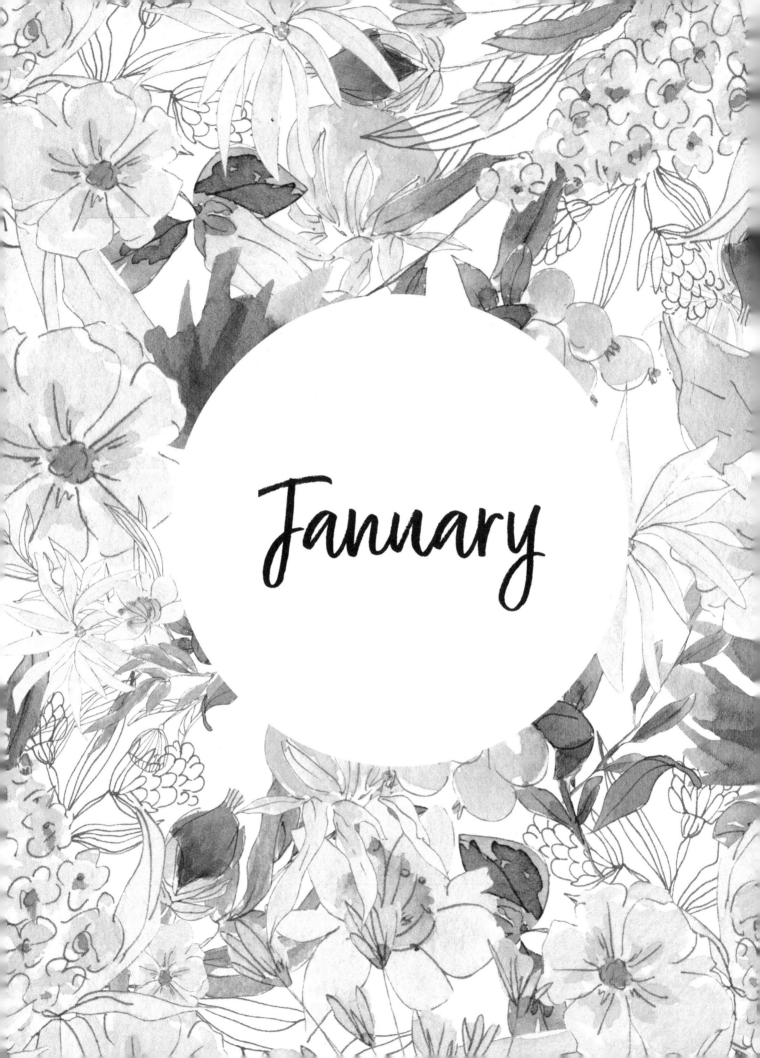

January

January

2021

MONTHLY GOALS

MONTHLY SNAPSHOT

TOP PRIORITIES

TASKS & NOTES

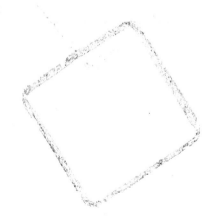

January

2021

SUNDAY	MONDAY	TUESDAY	WEDNESDAY
3	4	5	6
10	11	12	13
17	18	19	20
24	25	26	27

 I am **NOT DEFINED** by any limiting beliefs

January

2021

THURSDAY	FRIDAY	SATURDAY	TO-DO LIST
	1	2	○
			○
			○
			○
			○
7	8	9	○
			○
			○
			○
14	15	16	○
			○
			○
			○
			○
21	22	23	○
			○
			○
			○
			○
28	29	30	NOTES
		SUNDAY 31	

January TRACKER

Use this tracker to document your measurements and weight loss progress.

WEIGHT:	MEASUREMENT	NOTES
ARMS		
CHEST		
WAIST		
HIPS		
THIGHS		
BICEPS		
SHOULDERS		

LBS LOST/GAINED:	INCHES LOST:	OTHER:

2 WINS LAST MONTH

WHAT TO DO BETTER/IMPROVE THIS MONTH:

1	
2	
3	

3 THINGS I'VE LEARNED ABOUT MYSELF OVER THE LAST MONTH

Journaling / Notes / Brainstorming

WEEKLY *Food & Workout Tracker*

PLAN & TRACK YOUR MEALS & WORKOUTS

1 FRIDAY

MEALS

B _____

L _____

D _____

S

WATER ▢▢▢▢▢▢▢▢   FITNESS

2 SATURDAY

MEALS

B _____

L _____

D _____

S

WATER ▢▢▢▢▢▢▢▢   FITNESS

3 SUNDAY

MEALS

B _____

L _____

D _____

S

WATER ▢▢▢▢▢▢▢▢   FITNESS

4 MONDAY

MEALS

B _____

L _____

D _____

S

WATER ▢▢▢▢▢▢▢▢   FITNESS

5 TUESDAY

MEALS

B _____

L _____

D _____

S

WATER ▢▢▢▢▢▢▢▢   FITNESS

6 WEDNESDAY

MEALS

B _____

L _____

D _____

S

WATER ▢▢▢▢▢▢▢▢   FITNESS

7 THURSDAY

MEALS

B _____

L _____

D _____

S

WATER ▢▢▢▢▢▢▢▢   FITNESS

NOTES

WEEKLY *To-Do's*

1 Friday

HAPPINESS RATING: ☆☆☆☆☆

2 Saturday

HAPPINESS RATING: ☆☆☆☆☆

3 Sunday

HAPPINESS RATING: ☆☆☆☆☆

4 Monday

HAPPINESS RATING: ☆☆☆☆☆

5 Tuesday

HAPPINESS RATING: ☆☆☆☆☆

6 Wednesday

HAPPINESS RATING: ☆☆☆☆☆

7 Thursday

HAPPINESS RATING: ☆☆☆☆☆

WEEKLY *Food & Workout Tracker*

PLAN & TRACK YOUR MEAL & WORKOUTS

8 FRIDAY

MEALS

B _____

L _____

D _____

S

WATER ☐☐☐☐☐☐☐☐   FITNESS

9 SATURDAY

MEALS

B _____

L _____

D _____

S

WATER ☐☐☐☐☐☐☐☐   FITNESS

10 SUNDAY

MEALS

B _____

L _____

D _____

S

WATER ☐☐☐☐☐☐☐☐   FITNESS

11 MONDAY

MEALS

B _____

L _____

D _____

S

WATER ☐☐☐☐☐☐☐☐   FITNESS

12 TUESDAY

MEALS

B _____

L _____

D _____

S

WATER ☐☐☐☐☐☐☐☐   FITNESS

13 WEDNESDAY

MEALS

B _____

L _____

D _____

S

WATER ☐☐☐☐☐☐☐☐   FITNESS

14 THURSDAY

MEALS

B _____

L _____

D _____

S

WATER ☐☐☐☐☐☐☐☐   FITNESS

NOTES

WEEKLY To-Do's

8 Friday

....
....
....
....
....

HAPPINESS RATING: ☆☆☆☆☆

9 Saturday

....
....
....
....
....

HAPPINESS RATING: ☆☆☆☆☆

10 Sunday

....
....
....
....
....

HAPPINESS RATING: ☆☆☆☆☆

11 Monday

....
....
....
....
....

HAPPINESS RATING: ☆☆☆☆☆

12 Tuesday

....
....
....
....
....

HAPPINESS RATING: ☆☆☆☆☆

13 Wednesday

....
....
....
....
....

HAPPINESS RATING: ☆☆☆☆☆

14 Thursday

....
....
....

HAPPINESS RATING: ☆☆☆☆☆

WEEKLY *Food & Workout Tracker*

PLAN & TRACK YOUR MEALS & WORKOUTS

15 FRIDAY

MEALS

B _____

L _____

D _____

S

WATER ☐☐☐☐☐☐☐ FITNESS

16 SATURDAY

MEALS

B _____

L _____

D _____

S

WATER ☐☐☐☐☐☐☐ FITNESS

17 SUNDAY

MEALS

B _____

L _____

D _____

S

WATER ☐☐☐☐☐☐☐ FITNESS

18 MONDAY

MEALS

B _____

L _____

D _____

S

WATER ☐☐☐☐☐☐☐ FITNESS

19 TUESDAY

MEALS

B _____

L _____

D _____

S

WATER ☐☐☐☐☐☐☐ FITNESS

20 WEDNESDAY

MEALS

B _____

L _____

D _____

S

WATER ☐☐☐☐☐☐☐ FITNESS

21 THURSDAY

MEALS

B _____

L _____

D _____

S

WATER ☐☐☐☐☐☐☐ FITNESS

NOTES

WEEKLY To-Do's

15 Friday

....
....
....
....
....
....

HAPPINESS RATING: ☆☆☆☆☆

16 Saturday

....
....
....
....
....
....

HAPPINESS RATING: ☆☆☆☆☆

17 Sunday

....
....
....
....
....
....

HAPPINESS RATING: ☆☆☆☆☆

18 Monday

....
....
....
....
....
....

HAPPINESS RATING: ☆☆☆☆☆

19 Tuesday

....
....
....
....
....
....

HAPPINESS RATING: ☆☆☆☆☆

20 Wednesday

....
....
....
....
....
....

HAPPINESS RATING: ☆☆☆☆☆

21 Thursday

....
....
....

HAPPINESS RATING: ☆☆☆☆☆

WEEKLY *Food & Workout Tracker*

PLAN & TRACK YOUR MEALS & WORKOUTS

22 FRIDAY

MEALS

B _____

L _____

D _____

S

WATER ☐☐☐☐☐☐☐☐   FITNESS

23 SATURDAY

MEALS

B _____

L _____

D _____

S

WATER ☐☐☐☐☐☐☐☐   FITNESS

24 SUNDAY

MEALS

B _____

L _____

D _____

S

WATER ☐☐☐☐☐☐☐☐   FITNESS

25 MONDAY

MEALS

B _____

L _____

D _____

S

WATER ☐☐☐☐☐☐☐☐   FITNESS

26 TUESDAY

MEALS

B _____

L _____

D _____

S

WATER ☐☐☐☐☐☐☐☐   FITNESS

27 WEDNESDAY

MEALS

B _____

L _____

D _____

S

WATER ☐☐☐☐☐☐☐☐   FITNESS

28 THURSDAY

MEALS

B _____

L _____

D _____

S

WATER ☐☐☐☐☐☐☐☐   FITNESS

NOTES

WEEKLY *To-Do's*

22 Friday

....
....
....
....
....

HAPPINESS RATING: ☆☆☆☆☆

23 Saturday

....
....
....
....
....

HAPPINESS RATING: ☆☆☆☆☆

24 Sunday

....
....
....
....
....

HAPPINESS RATING: ☆☆☆☆☆

25 Monday

....
....
....
....
....

HAPPINESS RATING: ☆☆☆☆☆

26 Tuesday

....
....
....
....
....

HAPPINESS RATING: ☆☆☆☆☆

27 Wednesday

....
....
....
....
....

HAPPINESS RATING: ☆☆☆☆☆

28 Thursday

....
....
....

HAPPINESS RATING: ☆☆☆☆☆

WEEKLY *Food & Workout Tracker*

PLAN & TRACK YOUR MEALS & WORKOUTS

29 FRIDAY

MEALS

B _____

L _____

D _____

S

WATER 🥛🥛🥛🥛🥛🥛🥛🥛   FITNESS

30 SATURDAY

MEALS

B _____

L _____

D _____

S

WATER 🥛🥛🥛🥛🥛🥛🥛🥛   FITNESS

31 SUNDAY

MEALS

B _____

L _____

D _____

S

WATER 🥛🥛🥛🥛🥛🥛🥛🥛   FITNESS

NOTES

WEEKLY *To-Do's*

29 Friday

....
....
....
....
....
....

HAPPINESS RATING: ☆ ☆ ☆ ☆ ☆

30 Saturday

....
....
....
....
....
....

HAPPINESS RATING: ☆ ☆ ☆ ☆ ☆

31 Sunday

....
....
....
....
....
....

HAPPINESS RATING: ☆ ☆ ☆ ☆ ☆

Thoughts/notes about the month:

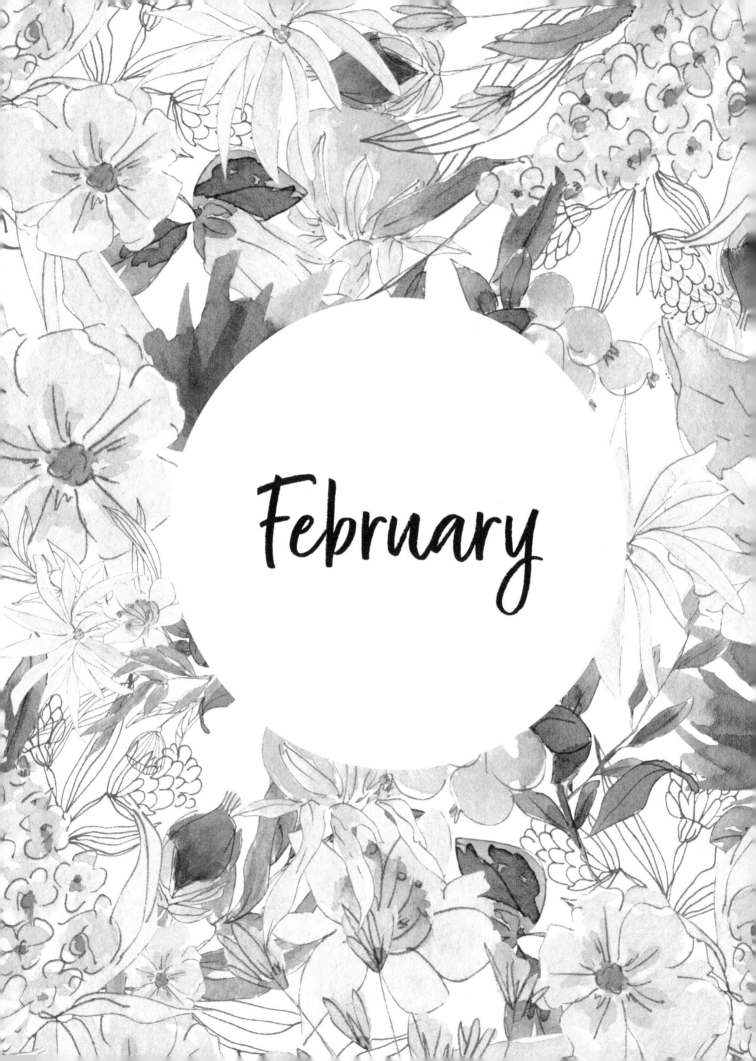

February

February

2021

MONTHLY SNAPSHOT

TOP PRIORITIES

TASKS & NOTES

February

SUNDAY	MONDAY	TUESDAY	WEDNESDAY
	1	2	3
7	8	9	10
14	15	16	17
21	22	23	24
28			

I am.... SOLUTION FOCUSED *not* PROBLEM FOCUSED

February

THURSDAY	FRIDAY	SATURDAY	TO-DO LIST
4	5	6	○
			○
			○
			○
			○
11	12	13	○
			○
			○
			○
18	19	20	○
			○
			○
			○
			○
25	26	27	○
			○
			○
			○
			○
			NOTES

February TRACKER

Use this tracker to document your measurements and weight loss progress.

WEIGHT:	MEASUREMENT	NOTES
ARMS		
CHEST		
WAIST		
HIPS		
THIGHS		
BICEPS		
SHOULDERS		

LBS LOST/GAINED:	INCHES LOST:	OTHER:

2 WINS LAST MONTH

WHAT TO DO BETTER/IMPROVE THIS MONTH:

1	
2	
3	

3 THINGS I'VE LEARNED ABOUT MYSELF OVER THE LAST MONTH

Journaling / Notes / Brainstorming

WEEKLY *Food & Workout Tracker*

PLAN & TRACK YOUR MEALS & WORKOUTS

1 MONDAY

MEALS

B

L

D

S

WATER ☐☐☐☐☐☐☐ FITNESS

2 TUESDAY

MEALS

B

L

D

S

WATER ☐☐☐☐☐☐☐ FITNESS

3 WEDNESDAY

MEALS

B

L

D

S

WATER ☐☐☐☐☐☐☐ FITNESS

4 THURSDAY

MEALS

B

L

D

S

WATER ☐☐☐☐☐☐☐ FITNESS

5 FRIDAY

MEALS

B

L

D

S

WATER ☐☐☐☐☐☐☐ FITNESS

6 SATURDAY

MEALS

B

L

D

S

WATER ☐☐☐☐☐☐☐ FITNESS

7 SUNDAY

MEALS

B

L

D

S

WATER ☐☐☐☐☐☐☐ FITNESS

NOTES

WEEKLY *To-Do's*

1 Monday

HAPPINESS RATING: ☆☆☆☆☆

2 Tuesday

HAPPINESS RATING: ☆☆☆☆☆

3 Wednesday

HAPPINESS RATING: ☆☆☆☆☆

4 Thursday

HAPPINESS RATING: ☆☆☆☆☆

5 Friday

HAPPINESS RATING: ☆☆☆☆☆

6 Saturday

HAPPINESS RATING: ☆☆☆☆☆

7 Sunday

HAPPINESS RATING: ☆☆☆☆☆

WEEKLY *Food & Workout Tracker*

PLAN & TRACK YOUR MEALS & WORKOUTS

8 MONDAY

MEALS

B _____

L _____

D _____

S

WATER ▢▢▢▢▢▢▢   FITNESS

9 TUESDAY

MEALS

B _____

L _____

D _____

S

WATER ▢▢▢▢▢▢▢   FITNESS

10 WEDNESDAY

MEALS

B _____

L _____

D _____

S

WATER ▢▢▢▢▢▢▢   FITNESS

11 THURSDAY

MEALS

B _____

L _____

D _____

S

WATER ▢▢▢▢▢▢▢   FITNESS

12 FRIDAY

MEALS

B _____

L _____

D _____

S

WATER ▢▢▢▢▢▢▢   FITNESS

13 SATURDAY

MEALS

B _____

L _____

D _____

S

WATER ▢▢▢▢▢▢▢   FITNESS

14 SUNDAY

MEALS

B _____

L _____

D _____

S

WATER ▢▢▢▢▢▢▢   FITNESS

NOTES

WEEKLY To-Do's

8 Monday

HAPPINESS RATING: ☆☆☆☆☆

9 Tuesday

HAPPINESS RATING: ☆☆☆☆☆

10 Wednesday

HAPPINESS RATING: ☆☆☆☆☆

11 Thursday

HAPPINESS RATING: ☆☆☆☆☆

12 Friday

HAPPINESS RATING: ☆☆☆☆☆

13 Saturday

HAPPINESS RATING: ☆☆☆☆☆

14 Sunday

HAPPINESS RATING: ☆☆☆☆☆

WEEKLY *Food & Workout Tracker*

PLAN & TRACK YOUR MEALS & WORKOUTS

15 MONDAY

MEALS

B _____
L _____
D _____
S _____

WATER ▢▢▢▢▢▢▢▢   FITNESS

16 TUESDAY

MEALS

B _____
L _____
D _____
S _____

WATER ▢▢▢▢▢▢▢▢   FITNESS

17 WEDNESDAY

MEALS

B _____
L _____
D _____
S _____

WATER ▢▢▢▢▢▢▢▢   FITNESS

18 THURSDAY

MEALS

B _____
L _____
D _____
S _____

WATER ▢▢▢▢▢▢▢▢   FITNESS

19 FRIDAY

MEALS

B _____
L _____
D _____
S _____

WATER ▢▢▢▢▢▢▢▢   FITNESS

20 SATURDAY

MEALS

B _____
L _____
D _____
S _____

WATER ▢▢▢▢▢▢▢▢   FITNESS

21 SUNDAY

MEALS

B _____
L _____
D _____
S _____

WATER ▢▢▢▢▢▢▢▢   FITNESS

NOTES

WEEKLY *To-Do's*

15 Monday

HAPPINESS RATING: ☆☆☆☆☆

16 Tuesday

HAPPINESS RATING: ☆☆☆☆☆

17 Wednesday

HAPPINESS RATING: ☆☆☆☆☆

18 Thursday

HAPPINESS RATING: ☆☆☆☆☆

19 Friday

HAPPINESS RATING: ☆☆☆☆☆

20 Saturday

HAPPINESS RATING: ☆☆☆☆☆

21 Sunday

HAPPINESS RATING: ☆☆☆☆☆

WEEKLY *Food & Workout Tracker*

PLAN & TRACK YOUR MEALS & WORKOUTS

22 MONDAY

MEALS

B _____
L _____
D _____
S

WATER ☐☐☐☐☐☐☐☐   FITNESS

23 TUESDAY

MEALS

B _____
L _____
D _____
S

WATER ☐☐☐☐☐☐☐☐   FITNESS

24 WEDNESDAY

MEALS

B _____
L _____
D _____
S

WATER ☐☐☐☐☐☐☐☐   FITNESS

25 THURSDAY

MEALS

B _____
L _____
D _____
S

WATER ☐☐☐☐☐☐☐☐   FITNESS

26 FRIDAY

MEALS

B _____
L _____
D _____
S

WATER ☐☐☐☐☐☐☐☐   FITNESS

27 SATURDAY

MEALS

B _____
L _____
D _____
S

WATER ☐☐☐☐☐☐☐☐   FITNESS

28 SUNDAY

MEALS

B _____
L _____
D _____
S

WATER ☐☐☐☐☐☐☐☐   FITNESS

NOTES

WEEKLY *To-Do's*

22 Monday

HAPPINESS RATING: ☆☆☆☆☆

23 Tuesday

HAPPINESS RATING: ☆☆☆☆☆

24 Wednesday

HAPPINESS RATING: ☆☆☆☆☆

25 Thursday

HAPPINESS RATING: ☆☆☆☆☆

26 Friday

HAPPINESS RATING: ☆☆☆☆☆

27 Saturday

HAPPINESS RATING: ☆☆☆☆☆

28 Sunday

HAPPINESS RATING: ☆☆☆☆☆

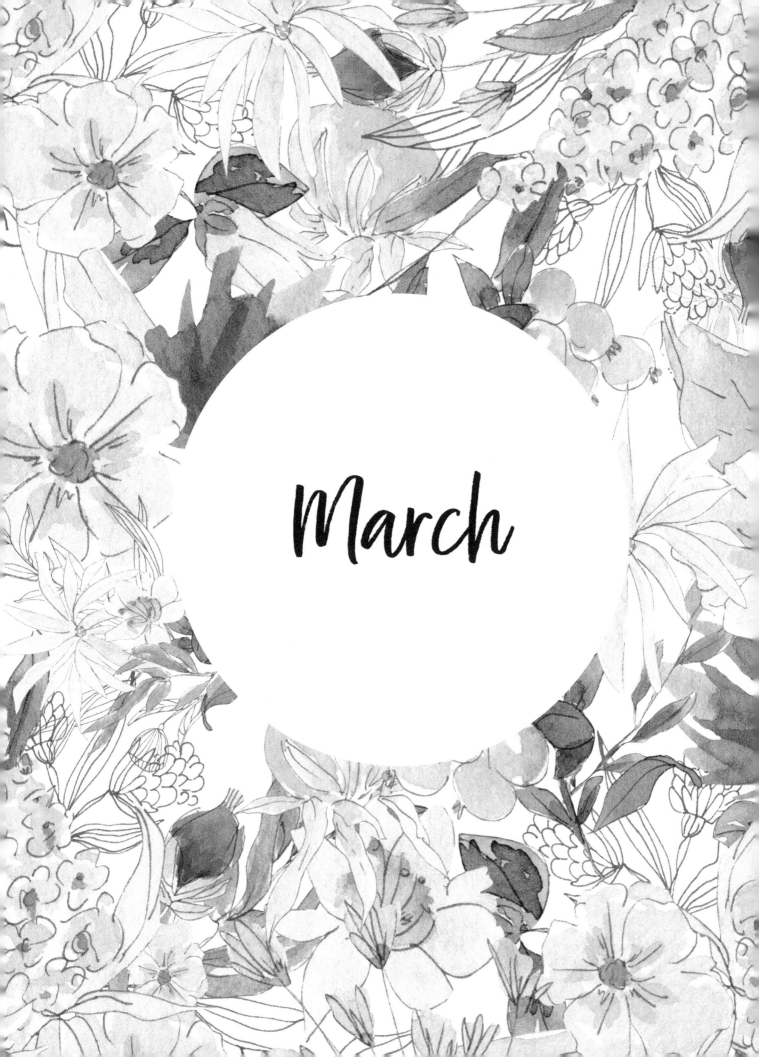

March

March

2021

Monthly Snapshot

Monthly Goals

Top Priorities

Tasks & Notes

March 2021

SUNDAY	MONDAY	TUESDAY	WEDNESDAY
	1	2	3
7	8	9	10
14	15	16	17
21	22	23	24
28	29	30	31

My thoughts & feelings are ⋛ **NOT** ⋚ **NECESSARILY** the truth.

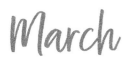

March

2021

THURSDAY	FRIDAY	SATURDAY	TO-DO LIST
4	5	6	○
			○
			○
			○
			○
11	12	13	○
			○
			○
			○
18	19	20	○
			○
			○
			○
			○
25	26	27	○
			○
			○
			○
			○
			NOTES

March TRACKER

Use this tracker to document your measurements and weight loss progress.

WEIGHT:	MEASUREMENT	NOTES
ARMS		
CHEST		
WAIST		
HIPS		
THIGHS		
BICEPS		
SHOULDERS		

LBS LOST/GAINED:	INCHES LOST:	OTHER:

2 WINS LAST MONTH

WHAT TO DO BETTER/IMPROVE THIS MONTH:

1
2
3

3 THINGS I'VE LEARNED ABOUT MYSELF OVER THE LAST MONTH

Journaling / Notes / Brainstorming

WEEKLY *Food & Workout Tracker*

PLAN & TRACK YOUR MEALS & WORKOUTS

1 MONDAY

MEALS

B _____

L _____

D _____

S _____

WATER ☐☐☐☐☐☐☐☐ FITNESS

2 TUESDAY

MEALS

B _____

L _____

D _____

S _____

WATER ☐☐☐☐☐☐☐☐ FITNESS

3 WEDNESDAY

MEALS

B _____

L _____

D _____

S _____

WATER ☐☐☐☐☐☐☐☐ FITNESS

4 THURSDAY

MEALS

B _____

L _____

D _____

S _____

WATER ☐☐☐☐☐☐☐☐ FITNESS

5 FRIDAY

MEALS

B _____

L _____

D _____

S _____

WATER ☐☐☐☐☐☐☐☐ FITNESS

6 SATURDAY

MEALS

B _____

L _____

D _____

S _____

WATER ☐☐☐☐☐☐☐☐ FITNESS

7 SUNDAY

MEALS

B _____

L _____

D _____

S _____

WATER ☐☐☐☐☐☐☐☐ FITNESS

NOTES

WEEKLY To-Do's

1 Monday

....
....
....
....
....

HAPPINESS RATING: ☆☆☆☆☆

2 Tuesday

....
....
....
....
....

HAPPINESS RATING: ☆☆☆☆☆

3 Wednesday

....
....
....
....
....

HAPPINESS RATING: ☆☆☆☆☆

4 Thursday

....
....
....
....
....

HAPPINESS RATING: ☆☆☆☆☆

5 Friday

....
....
....
....
....

HAPPINESS RATING: ☆☆☆☆☆

6 Saturday

....
....
....
....
....

HAPPINESS RATING: ☆☆☆☆☆

7 Sunday

....
....
....

HAPPINESS RATING: ☆☆☆☆☆

WEEKLY *Food & Workout Tracker*

PLAN & TRACK YOUR MEALS & WORKOUTS

8 MONDAY

MEALS

B

L

D

S

WATER ▢▢▢▢▢▢▢   FITNESS

9 TUESDAY

MEALS

B

L

D

S

WATER ▢▢▢▢▢▢▢   FITNESS

10 WEDNESDAY

MEALS

B

L

D

S

WATER ▢▢▢▢▢▢▢   FITNESS

11 THURSDAY

MEALS

B

L

D

S

WATER ▢▢▢▢▢▢▢   FITNESS

12 FRIDAY

MEALS

B

L

D

S

WATER ▢▢▢▢▢▢▢   FITNESS

13 SATURDAY

MEALS

B

L

D

S

WATER ▢▢▢▢▢▢▢   FITNESS

14 SUNDAY

MEALS

B

L

D

S

WATER ▢▢▢▢▢▢▢   FITNESS

NOTES

WEEKLY *To-Do's*

8 Monday

....
....
....
....
....

HAPPINESS RATING: ☆☆☆☆☆

9 Tuesday

....
....
....
....
....

HAPPINESS RATING: ☆☆☆☆☆

10 Wednesday

....
....
....
....
....

HAPPINESS RATING: ☆☆☆☆☆

11 Thursday

....
....
....
....
....

HAPPINESS RATING: ☆☆☆☆☆

12 Friday

....
....
....
....
....

HAPPINESS RATING: ☆☆☆☆☆

13 Saturday

....
....
....
....
....

HAPPINESS RATING: ☆☆☆☆☆

14 Sunday

....
....
....

HAPPINESS RATING: ☆☆☆☆☆

WEEKLY *Food & Workout Tracker*

PLAN & TRACK YOUR MEALS & WORKOUTS

15 MONDAY

MEALS

B _____

L _____

D _____

S

WATER ▢▢▢▢▢▢▢   **FITNESS**

16 TUESDAY

MEALS

B _____

L _____

D _____

S

WATER ▢▢▢▢▢▢▢   **FITNESS**

17 WEDNESDAY

MEALS

B _____

L _____

D _____

S

WATER ▢▢▢▢▢▢▢   **FITNESS**

18 THURSDAY

MEALS

B _____

L _____

D _____

S

WATER ▢▢▢▢▢▢▢   **FITNESS**

19 FRIDAY

MEALS

B _____

L _____

D _____

S

WATER ▢▢▢▢▢▢▢   **FITNESS**

20 SATURDAY

MEALS

B _____

L _____

D _____

S

WATER ▢▢▢▢▢▢▢   **FITNESS**

21 SUNDAY

MEALS

B _____

L _____

D _____

S

WATER ▢▢▢▢▢▢▢   **FITNESS**

NOTES

WEEKLY *To-Do's*

15 Monday

HAPPINESS RATING: ☆☆☆☆☆

16 Tuesday

HAPPINESS RATING: ☆☆☆☆☆

17 Wednesday

HAPPINESS RATING: ☆☆☆☆☆

18 Thursday

HAPPINESS RATING: ☆☆☆☆☆

19 Friday

HAPPINESS RATING: ☆☆☆☆☆

20 Saturday

HAPPINESS RATING: ☆☆☆☆☆

21 Sunday

HAPPINESS RATING: ☆☆☆☆☆

WEEKLY *Food & Workout Tracker*

PLAN & TRACK YOUR MEALS & WORKOUTS

22 MONDAY

MEALS

B

L

D

S

WATER ⬜⬜⬜⬜⬜⬜⬜   FITNESS

23 TUESDAY

MEALS

B

L

D

S

WATER ⬜⬜⬜⬜⬜⬜⬜   FITNESS

24 WEDNESDAY

MEALS

B

L

D

S

WATER ⬜⬜⬜⬜⬜⬜⬜   FITNESS

25 THURSDAY

MEALS

B

L

D

S

WATER ⬜⬜⬜⬜⬜⬜⬜   FITNESS

26 FRIDAY

MEALS

B

L

D

S

WATER ⬜⬜⬜⬜⬜⬜⬜   FITNESS

27 SATURDAY

MEALS

B

L

D

S

WATER ⬜⬜⬜⬜⬜⬜⬜   FITNESS

28 SUNDAY

MEALS

B

L

D

S

WATER ⬜⬜⬜⬜⬜⬜⬜   FITNESS

NOTES

WEEKLY *To-Do's*

22 Monday

....
....
....
....
....

HAPPINESS RATING: ☆☆☆☆☆

23 Tuesday

....
....
....
....
....

HAPPINESS RATING: ☆☆☆☆☆

24 Wednesday

....
....
....
....
....

HAPPINESS RATING: ☆☆☆☆☆

25 Thursday

....
....
....
....
....

HAPPINESS RATING: ☆☆☆☆☆

26 Friday

....
....
....
....
....

HAPPINESS RATING: ☆☆☆☆☆

27 Saturday

....
....
....
....
....

HAPPINESS RATING: ☆☆☆☆☆

28 Sunday

....
....

HAPPINESS RATING: ☆☆☆☆☆

WEEKLY *Food & Workout Tracker*

PLAN & TRACK YOUR MEALS & WORKOUTS

29 MONDAY

MEALS

B _____

L _____

D _____

S

WATER ▢▢▢▢▢▢▢▢ **FITNESS**

30 TUESDAY

MEALS

B _____

L _____

D _____

S

WATER ▢▢▢▢▢▢▢▢ **FITNESS**

31 WEDNESDAY

MEALS

B _____

L _____

D _____

S

WATER ▢▢▢▢▢▢▢▢ **FITNESS**

NOTES

WEEKLY *To-Do's*

29 Monday

....
....
....
....
....
....

HAPPINESS RATING: ☆☆☆☆☆

30 Tuesday

....
....
....
....
....
....

HAPPINESS RATING: ☆☆☆☆☆

31 Wednesday

....
....
....
....
....
....

HAPPINESS RATING: ☆☆☆☆☆

Thoughts/notes about the month:

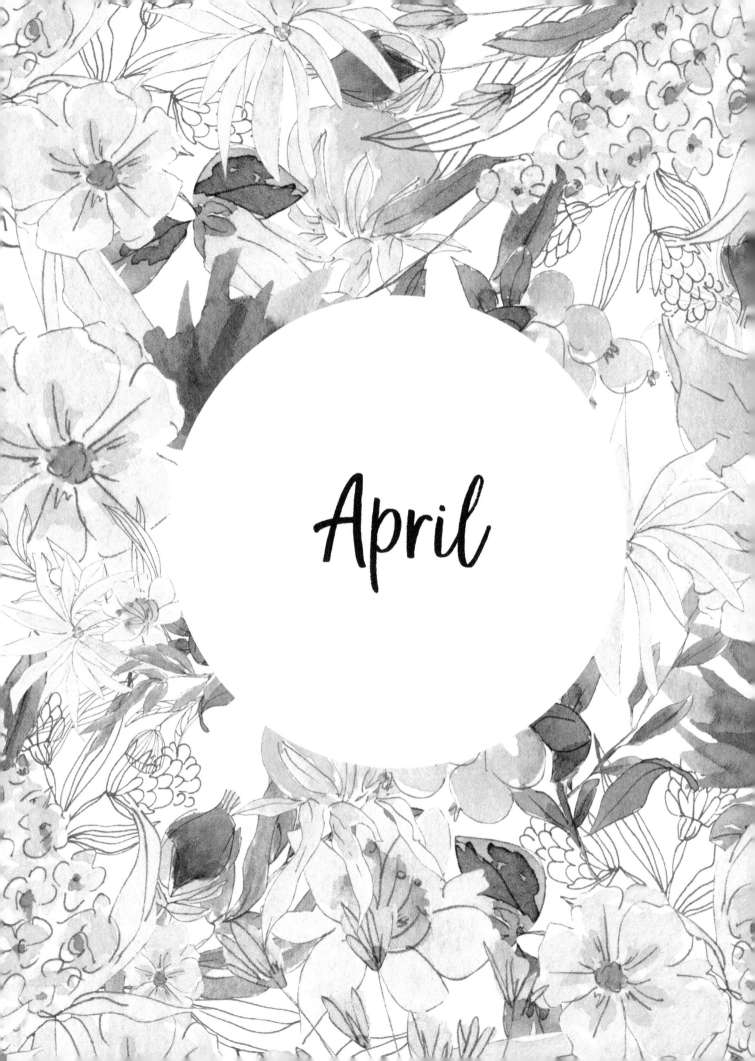

April

April

2021

Monthly Goals

Monthly Snapshot

Top Priorities

Tasks & Notes

April

SUNDAY	MONDAY	TUESDAY	WEDNESDAY
4	5	6	7
11	12	13	14
18	19	20	21
25	26	27	28

I am **PATIENT** with myself on my path to wellness.

April

2021

THURSDAY	FRIDAY	SATURDAY	TO-DO LIST
1	2	3	○
			○
			○
			○
			○
8	9	10	○
			○
			○
			○
15	16	17	○
			○
			○
			○
			○
22	23	24	○
			○
			○
			○
			○
29	30		NOTES

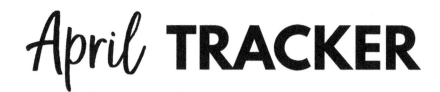

April TRACKER

Use this tracker to document your measurements and weight loss progress.

WEIGHT:	MEASUREMENT	NOTES
ARMS		
CHEST		
WAIST		
HIPS		
THIGHS		
BICEPS		
SHOULDERS		

LBS LOST/GAINED:	INCHES LOST:	OTHER:

2 WINS LAST MONTH

WHAT TO DO BETTER/IMPROVE THIS MONTH:

1	
2	
3	

3 THINGS I'VE LEARNED ABOUT MYSELF OVER THE LAST MONTH

WEEKLY *Food & Workout Tracker*

PLAN & TRACK YOUR MEALS & WORKOUTS

1 THURSDAY

MEALS

B _____

L _____

D _____

S _____

WATER ☐☐☐☐☐☐☐☐   **FITNESS**

2 FRIDAY

MEALS

B _____

L _____

D _____

S _____

WATER ☐☐☐☐☐☐☐☐   **FITNESS**

3 SATURDAY

MEALS

B _____

L _____

D _____

S _____

WATER ☐☐☐☐☐☐☐☐   **FITNESS**

4 SUNDAY

MEALS

B _____

L _____

D _____

S _____

WATER ☐☐☐☐☐☐☐☐   **FITNESS**

5 MONDAY

MEALS

B _____

L _____

D _____

S _____

WATER ☐☐☐☐☐☐☐☐   **FITNESS**

6 TUESDAY

MEALS

B _____

L _____

D _____

S _____

WATER ☐☐☐☐☐☐☐☐   **FITNESS**

7 WEDNESDAY

MEALS

B _____

L _____

D _____

S _____

WATER ☐☐☐☐☐☐☐☐   **FITNESS**

NOTES

WEEKLY *To-Do's*

1 Thursday

HAPPINESS RATING: ☆☆☆☆☆

2 Friday

HAPPINESS RATING: ☆☆☆☆☆

3 Saturday

HAPPINESS RATING: ☆☆☆☆☆

4 Sunday

HAPPINESS RATING: ☆☆☆☆☆

5 Monday

HAPPINESS RATING: ☆☆☆☆☆

6 Tuesday

HAPPINESS RATING: ☆☆☆☆☆

7 Wednesday

HAPPINESS RATING: ☆☆☆☆☆

WEEKLY *Food & Workout Tracker*

PLAN & TRACK YOUR MEALS & WORKOUTS

8 THURSDAY

MEALS

B _____

L _____

D _____

S

WATER ☐☐☐☐☐☐☐☐   FITNESS

9 FRIDAY

MEALS

B _____

L _____

D _____

S

WATER ☐☐☐☐☐☐☐☐   FITNESS

10 SATURDAY

MEALS

B _____

L _____

D _____

S

WATER ☐☐☐☐☐☐☐☐   FITNESS

11 SUNDAY

MEALS

B _____

L _____

D _____

S

WATER ☐☐☐☐☐☐☐☐   FITNESS

12 MONDAY

MEALS

B _____

L _____

D _____

S

WATER ☐☐☐☐☐☐☐☐   FITNESS

13 TUESDAY

MEALS

B _____

L _____

D _____

S

WATER ☐☐☐☐☐☐☐☐   FITNESS

14 WEDNESDAY

MEALS

B _____

L _____

D _____

S

WATER ☐☐☐☐☐☐☐☐   FITNESS

NOTES

WEEKLY *To-Do's*

8 Thursday

....
....
....
....
....

HAPPINESS RATING: ☆☆☆☆☆

9 Friday

....
....
....
....
....

HAPPINESS RATING: ☆☆☆☆☆

10 Saturday

....
....
....
....
....

HAPPINESS RATING: ☆☆☆☆☆

11 Sunday

....
....
....
....
....

HAPPINESS RATING: ☆☆☆☆☆

12 Monday

....
....
....
....
....

HAPPINESS RATING: ☆☆☆☆☆

13 Tuesday

....
....
....
....
....

HAPPINESS RATING: ☆☆☆☆☆

14 Wednesday

....
....

HAPPINESS RATING: ☆☆☆☆☆

WEEKLY *Food & Workout Tracker*

PLAN & TRACK YOUR MEALS & WORKOUTS

15 THURSDAY

MEALS

B _____

L _____

D _____

S

WATER ▢▢▢▢▢▢▢▢   FITNESS

16 FRIDAY

MEALS

B _____

L _____

D _____

S

WATER ▢▢▢▢▢▢▢▢   FITNESS

17 SATURDAY

MEALS

B _____

L _____

D _____

S

WATER ▢▢▢▢▢▢▢▢   FITNESS

18 SUNDAY

MEALS

B _____

L _____

D _____

S

WATER ▢▢▢▢▢▢▢▢   FITNESS

19 MONDAY

MEALS

B _____

L _____

D _____

S

WATER ▢▢▢▢▢▢▢▢   FITNESS

20 TUESDAY

MEALS

B _____

L _____

D _____

S

WATER ▢▢▢▢▢▢▢▢   FITNESS

21 WEDNESDAY

MEALS

B _____

L _____

D _____

S

WATER ▢▢▢▢▢▢▢▢   FITNESS

NOTES

WEEKLY *To-Do's*

15 Thursday

....
....
....
....
....
....

HAPPINESS RATING: ☆☆☆☆☆

16 Friday

....
....
....
....
....
....

HAPPINESS RATING: ☆☆☆☆☆

17 Saturday

....
....
....
....
....
....

HAPPINESS RATING: ☆☆☆☆☆

18 Sunday

....
....
....
....
....

HAPPINESS RATING: ☆☆☆☆☆

19 Monday

....
....
....
....
....

HAPPINESS RATING: ☆☆☆☆☆

20 Tuesday

....
....
....
....
....

HAPPINESS RATING: ☆☆☆☆☆

21 Wednesday

....
....
....

HAPPINESS RATING: ☆☆☆☆☆

WEEKLY *Food & Workout Tracker*

PLAN & TRACK YOUR MEALS & WORKOUTS

22 THURSDAY

MEALS

B _____

L _____

D _____

S

WATER ☐☐☐☐☐☐☐ FITNESS

23 FRIDAY

MEALS

B _____

L _____

D _____

S

WATER ☐☐☐☐☐☐☐ FITNESS

24 SATURDAY

MEALS

B _____

L _____

D _____

S

WATER ☐☐☐☐☐☐☐ FITNESS

25 SUNDAY

MEALS

B _____

L _____

D _____

S

WATER ☐☐☐☐☐☐☐ FITNESS

26 MONDAY

MEALS

B _____

L _____

D _____

S

WATER ☐☐☐☐☐☐☐ FITNESS

27 TUESDAY

MEALS

B _____

L _____

D _____

S

WATER ☐☐☐☐☐☐☐ FITNESS

28 WEDNESDAY

MEALS

B _____

L _____

D _____

S

WATER ☐☐☐☐☐☐☐ FITNESS

NOTES

WEEKLY *To-Do's*

22 Thursday

HAPPINESS RATING: ☆☆☆☆☆

23 Friday

HAPPINESS RATING: ☆☆☆☆☆

24 Saturday

HAPPINESS RATING: ☆☆☆☆☆

25 Sunday

HAPPINESS RATING: ☆☆☆☆☆

26 Monday

HAPPINESS RATING: ☆☆☆☆☆

27 Tuesday

HAPPINESS RATING: ☆☆☆☆☆

28 Wednesday

HAPPINESS RATING: ☆☆☆☆☆

WEEKLY *Food & Workout Tracker*

PLAN & TRACK YOUR MEALS & WORKOUTS

29 THURSDAY

MEALS

B _____

L _____

D _____

S

WATER ▢▢▢▢▢▢▢ **FITNESS**

30 FRIDAY

MEALS

B _____

L _____

D _____

S

WATER ▢▢▢▢▢▢▢ **FITNESS**

NOTES

WEEKLY *To-Do's*

29 Thursday

....
....
....
....
....
....
....

HAPPINESS RATING: ☆ ☆ ☆ ☆ ☆

30 Friday

....
....
....
....
....
....
....

HAPPINESS RATING: ☆ ☆ ☆ ☆ ☆

Thoughts/notes about the month:

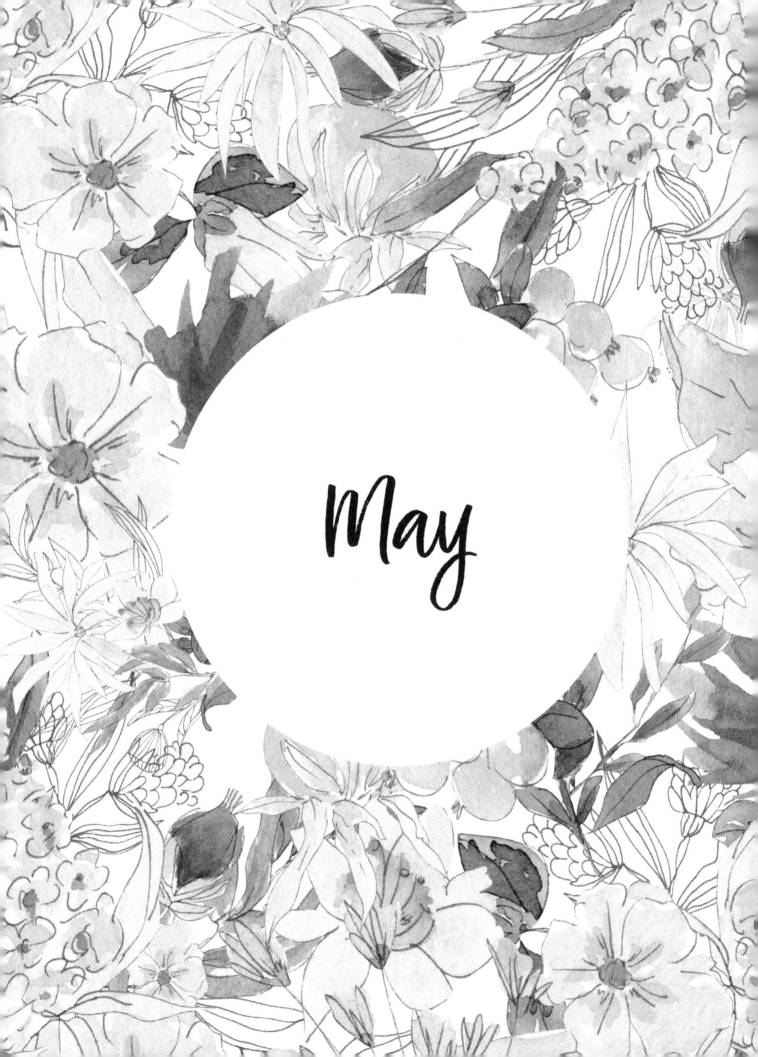

May

May

2021

MONTHLY SNAPSHOT

TOP PRIORITIES

TASKS & NOTES

May

2021

SUNDAY	MONDAY	TUESDAY	WEDNESDAY
2	3	4	5
9	10	11	12
16	17	18	19
23 / 30	24 / 31	25	26

I have been 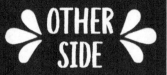 HERE BEFORE and I came out on the OTHER SIDE

May

2021

THURSDAY	FRIDAY	SATURDAY	TO-DO LIST
		1	○
			○
			○
			○
			○
6	7	8	○
			○
			○
			○
13	14	15	○
			○
			○
			○
			○
20	21	22	○
			○
			○
			○
			○
27	28	29	NOTES

May TRACKER

Use this tracker to document your measurements and weight loss progress.

WEIGHT:		MEASUREMENT	NOTES
	ARMS		
	CHEST		
	WAIST		
	HIPS		
	THIGHS		
	BICEPS		
	SHOULDERS		

LBS LOST/GAINED:	INCHES LOST:	OTHER:

2 WINS LAST MONTH

WHAT TO DO BETTER/IMPROVE THIS MONTH:

1	
2	
3	

3 THINGS I'VE LEARNED ABOUT MYSELF OVER THE LAST MONTH

Journaling / Notes / Brainstorming

WEEKLY *Food & Workout Tracker*

PLAN & TRACK YOUR MEALS & WORKOUTS

1 SATURDAY

MEALS

B

L

D

S

WATER ▢▢▢▢▢▢▢ FITNESS

2 SUNDAY

MEALS

B

L

D

S

WATER ▢▢▢▢▢▢▢ FITNESS

3 MONDAY

MEALS

B

L

D

S

WATER ▢▢▢▢▢▢▢ FITNESS

4 TUESDAY

MEALS

B

L

D

S

WATER ▢▢▢▢▢▢▢ FITNESS

5 WEDNESDAY

MEALS

B

L

D

S

WATER ▢▢▢▢▢▢▢ FITNESS

6 THURSDAY

MEALS

B

L

D

S

WATER ▢▢▢▢▢▢▢ FITNESS

7 FRIDAY

MEALS

B

L

D

S

WATER ▢▢▢▢▢▢▢ FITNESS

NOTES

WEEKLY To-Do's

1 Saturday

HAPPINESS RATING: ☆☆☆☆☆

2 Sunday

HAPPINESS RATING: ☆☆☆☆☆

3 Monday

HAPPINESS RATING: ☆☆☆☆☆

4 Tuesday

HAPPINESS RATING: ☆☆☆☆☆

5 Wednesday

HAPPINESS RATING: ☆☆☆☆☆

6 Thursday

HAPPINESS RATING: ☆☆☆☆☆

7 Friday

HAPPINESS RATING: ☆☆☆☆☆

WEEKLY *Food & Workout Tracker*

PLAN & TRACK YOUR MEALS & WORKOUTS

8 SATURDAY

MEALS

B _____
L _____
D _____
S

WATER ▢▢▢▢▢▢▢   FITNESS

9 SUNDAY

MEALS

B _____
L _____
D _____
S

WATER ▢▢▢▢▢▢▢   FITNESS

10 MONDAY

MEALS

B _____
L _____
D _____
S

WATER ▢▢▢▢▢▢▢   FITNESS

11 TUESDAY

MEALS

B _____
L _____
D _____
S

WATER ▢▢▢▢▢▢▢   FITNESS

12 WEDNESDAY

MEALS

B _____
L _____
D _____
S

WATER ▢▢▢▢▢▢▢   FITNESS

13 THURSDAY

MEALS

B _____
L _____
D _____
S

WATER ▢▢▢▢▢▢▢   FITNESS

14 FRIDAY

MEALS

B _____
L _____
D _____
S

WATER ▢▢▢▢▢▢▢   FITNESS

NOTES

WEEKLY *To-Do's*

8 Saturday

....
....
....
....
....

HAPPINESS RATING: ☆☆☆☆☆

9 Sunday

....
....
....
....
....

HAPPINESS RATING: ☆☆☆☆☆

10 Monday

....
....
....
....
....

HAPPINESS RATING: ☆☆☆☆☆

11 Tuesday

....
....
....
....
....

HAPPINESS RATING: ☆☆☆☆☆

12 Wednesday

....
....
....
....
....

HAPPINESS RATING: ☆☆☆☆☆

13 Thursday

....
....
....
....
....

HAPPINESS RATING: ☆☆☆☆☆

14 Friday

....
....

HAPPINESS RATING: ☆☆☆☆☆

WEEKLY *Food & Workout Tracker*

PLAN & TRACK YOUR MEALS & WORKOUTS

15 SATURDAY

MEALS

B _____

L _____

D _____

S

WATER ☐☐☐☐☐☐☐☐   FITNESS

16 SUNDAY

MEALS

B _____

L _____

D _____

S

WATER ☐☐☐☐☐☐☐☐   FITNESS

17 MONDAY

MEALS

B _____

L _____

D _____

S

WATER ☐☐☐☐☐☐☐☐   FITNESS

18 TUESDAY

MEALS

B _____

L _____

D _____

S

WATER ☐☐☐☐☐☐☐☐   FITNESS

19 WEDNESDAY

MEALS

B _____

L _____

D _____

S

WATER ☐☐☐☐☐☐☐☐   FITNESS

20 THURSDAY

MEALS

B _____

L _____

D _____

S

WATER ☐☐☐☐☐☐☐☐   FITNESS

21 FRIDAY

MEALS

B _____

L _____

D _____

S

WATER ☐☐☐☐☐☐☐☐   FITNESS

NOTES

WEEKLY *To-Do's*

15 Saturday

....
....
....
....
....
....

HAPPINESS RATING: ☆☆☆☆☆

16 Sunday

....
....
....
....
....
....

HAPPINESS RATING: ☆☆☆☆☆

17 Monday

....
....
....
....
....
....

HAPPINESS RATING: ☆☆☆☆☆

18 Tuesday

....
....
....
....
....
....

HAPPINESS RATING: ☆☆☆☆☆

19 Wednesday

....
....
....
....
....
....

HAPPINESS RATING: ☆☆☆☆☆

20 Thursday

....
....
....
....
....
....

HAPPINESS RATING: ☆☆☆☆☆

21 Friday

....
....
....

HAPPINESS RATING: ☆☆☆☆☆

WEEKLY *Food & Workout Tracker*

PLAN & TRACK YOUR MEALS & WORKOUTS

22 SATURDAY

MEALS

B _____

L _____

D _____

S _____

WATER ⬜⬜⬜⬜⬜⬜⬜ FITNESS

23 SUNDAY

MEALS

B _____

L _____

D _____

S _____

WATER ⬜⬜⬜⬜⬜⬜⬜ FITNESS

24 MONDAY

MEALS

B _____

L _____

D _____

S _____

WATER ⬜⬜⬜⬜⬜⬜⬜ FITNESS

25 TUESDAY

MEALS

B _____

L _____

D _____

S _____

WATER ⬜⬜⬜⬜⬜⬜⬜ FITNESS

26 WEDNESDAY

MEALS

B _____

L _____

D _____

S _____

WATER ⬜⬜⬜⬜⬜⬜⬜ FITNESS

27 THURSDAY

MEALS

B _____

L _____

D _____

S _____

WATER ⬜⬜⬜⬜⬜⬜⬜ FITNESS

28 FRIDAY

MEALS

B _____

L _____

D _____

S _____

WATER ⬜⬜⬜⬜⬜⬜⬜ FITNESS

NOTES

WEEKLY *To-Do's*

22 Saturday

....
....
....
....
....

HAPPINESS RATING: ☆☆☆☆☆

23 Sunday

....
....
....
....
....

HAPPINESS RATING: ☆☆☆☆☆

24 Monday

....
....
....
....
....

HAPPINESS RATING: ☆☆☆☆☆

25 Tuesday

....
....
....
....
....

HAPPINESS RATING: ☆☆☆☆☆

26 Wednesday

....
....
....
....
....

HAPPINESS RATING: ☆☆☆☆☆

27 Thursday

....
....
....
....
....

HAPPINESS RATING: ☆☆☆☆☆

28 Friday

....
....
....

HAPPINESS RATING: ☆☆☆☆☆

WEEKLY *Food & Workout Tracker*

PLAN & TRACK YOUR MEALS & WORKOUTS

29 SATURDAY

MEALS

B _____

L _____

D _____

S

WATER ☐☐☐☐☐☐☐   FITNESS

30 SUNDAY

MEALS

B _____

L _____

D _____

S

WATER ☐☐☐☐☐☐☐   FITNESS

31 MONDAY

MEALS

B _____

L _____

D _____

S

WATER ☐☐☐☐☐☐☐   FITNESS

NOTES

WEEKLY *To-Do's*

29 Saturday

....
....
....
....
....
....
....

HAPPINESS
RATING: ☆☆☆☆☆

30 Sunday

....
....
....
....
....
....

HAPPINESS
RATING: ☆☆☆☆☆

31 Monday

....
....
....
....
....
....

HAPPINESS
RATING: ☆☆☆☆☆

Thoughts/notes about the month:

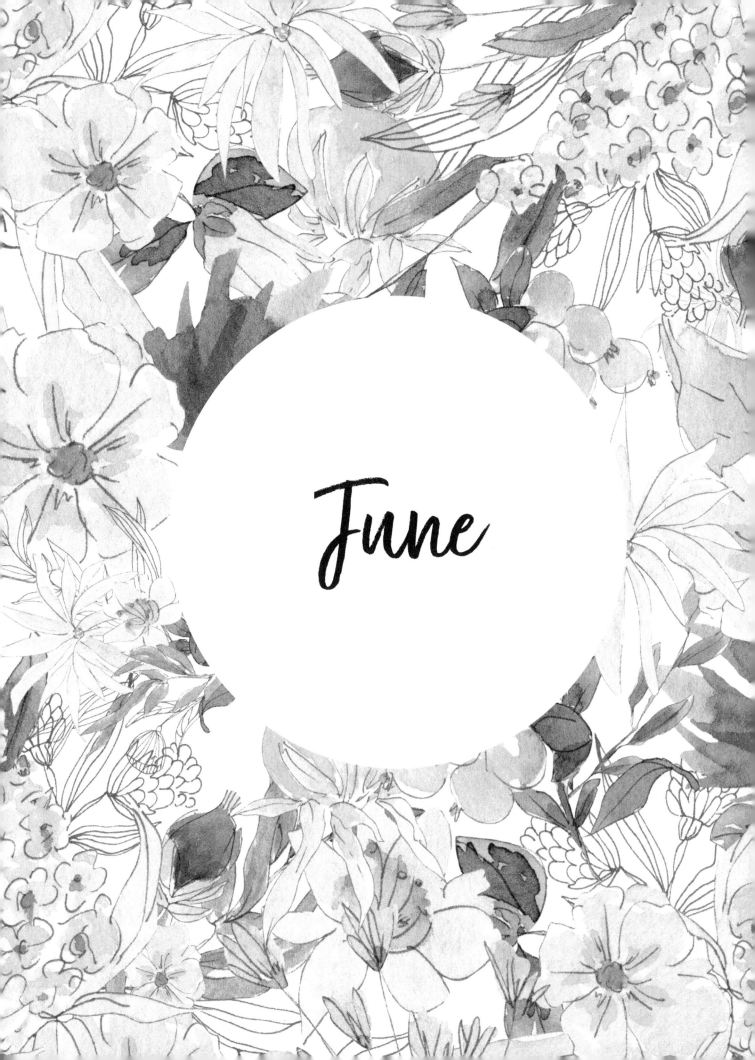

June

June

2021

Monthly Snapshot

Top Priorities

Monthly Goals

Tasks & Notes

June

SUNDAY	MONDAY	TUESDAY	WEDNESDAY
		1	2
6	7	8	9
13	14	15	16
20	21	22	23
27	28	29	30

I choose *Progress* **PROGRESS** *Over* **PERFECTION**

June

THURSDAY	FRIDAY	SATURDAY	TO-DO LIST
3	4	5	○
			○
			○
			○
			○
10	11	12	○
			○
			○
			○
17	18	19	○
			○
			○
			○
			○
24	25	26	○
			○
			○
			○
			○
			NOTES

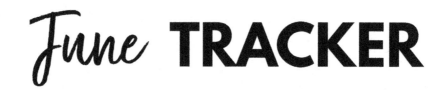

June TRACKER

Use this tracker to document your measurements and weight loss progress.

WEIGHT:	MEASUREMENT	NOTES
ARMS		
CHEST		
WAIST		
HIPS		
THIGHS		
BICEPS		
SHOULDERS		

LBS LOST/GAINED:	INCHES LOST:	OTHER:

2 WINS LAST MONTH

WHAT TO DO BETTER/IMPROVE THIS MONTH:

1
2
3

3 THINGS I'VE LEARNED ABOUT MYSELF OVER THE LAST MONTH

Journaling / Notes / Brainstorming

WEEKLY *Food & Workout Tracker*

PLAN & TRACK YOUR MEALS & WORKOUTS

1   TUESDAY

MEALS

B _____
L _____
D _____
S

WATER ☐☐☐☐☐☐☐☐   FITNESS

2   WEDNESDAY

MEALS

B _____
L _____
D _____
S

WATER ☐☐☐☐☐☐☐☐   FITNESS

3   THURSDAY

MEALS

B _____
L _____
D _____
S

WATER ☐☐☐☐☐☐☐☐   FITNESS

4   FRIDAY

MEALS

B _____
L _____
D _____
S

WATER ☐☐☐☐☐☐☐☐   FITNESS

5   SATURDAY

MEALS

B _____
L _____
D _____
S

WATER ☐☐☐☐☐☐☐☐   FITNESS

6   SUNDAY

MEALS

B _____
L _____
D _____
S

WATER ☐☐☐☐☐☐☐☐   FITNESS

7   MONDAY

MEALS

B _____
L _____
D _____
S

WATER ☐☐☐☐☐☐☐☐   FITNESS

NOTES

WEEKLY To-Do's

1 Tuesday

....
....
....
....
....

HAPPINESS RATING: ☆☆☆☆☆

2 Wednesday

....
....
....
....
....

HAPPINESS RATING: ☆☆☆☆☆

3 Thursday

....
....
....
....
....

HAPPINESS RATING: ☆☆☆☆☆

4 Friday

....
....
....
....
....

HAPPINESS RATING: ☆☆☆☆☆

5 Saturday

....
....
....
....
....

HAPPINESS RATING: ☆☆☆☆☆

6 Sunday

....
....
....
....
....

HAPPINESS RATING: ☆☆☆☆☆

7 Monday

....
....
....

HAPPINESS RATING: ☆☆☆☆☆

WEEKLY *Food & Workout Tracker*

PLAN & TRACK YOUR MEALS & WORKOUTS

8 TUESDAY

MEALS

B _____

L _____

D _____

S

WATER ▢▢▢▢▢▢▢▢   FITNESS

9 WEDNESDAY

MEALS

B _____

L _____

D _____

S

WATER ▢▢▢▢▢▢▢▢   FITNESS

10 THURSDAY

MEALS

B _____

L _____

D _____

S

WATER ▢▢▢▢▢▢▢▢   FITNESS

11 FRIDAY

MEALS

B _____

L _____

D _____

S

WATER ▢▢▢▢▢▢▢▢   FITNESS

12 SATURDAY

MEALS

B _____

L _____

D _____

S

WATER ▢▢▢▢▢▢▢▢   FITNESS

13 SUNDAY

MEALS

B _____

L _____

D _____

S

WATER ▢▢▢▢▢▢▢▢   FITNESS

14 MONDAY

MEALS

B _____

L _____

D _____

S

WATER ▢▢▢▢▢▢▢▢   FITNESS

NOTES

WEEKLY *To-Do's*

8 Tuesday

....
....
....
....
....

HAPPINESS RATING: ☆☆☆☆☆

9 Wednesday

....
....
....
....
....

HAPPINESS RATING: ☆☆☆☆☆

10 Thursday

....
....
....
....
....

HAPPINESS RATING: ☆☆☆☆☆

11 Friday

....
....
....
....
....

HAPPINESS RATING: ☆☆☆☆☆

12 Saturday

....
....
....
....
....

HAPPINESS RATING: ☆☆☆☆☆

13 Sunday

....
....
....
....
....

HAPPINESS RATING: ☆☆☆☆☆

14 Monday

....
....
....

HAPPINESS RATING: ☆☆☆☆☆

WEEKLY *Food & Workout Tracker*

PLAN & TRACK YOUR MEALS & WORKOUTS

15 TUESDAY

MEALS

B _____

L _____

D _____

S

WATER ▢▢▢▢▢▢▢ FITNESS

16 WEDNESDAY

MEALS

B _____

L _____

D _____

S

WATER ▢▢▢▢▢▢▢ FITNESS

17 THURSDAY

MEALS

B _____

L _____

D _____

S

WATER ▢▢▢▢▢▢▢ FITNESS

18 FRIDAY

MEALS

B _____

L _____

D _____

S

WATER ▢▢▢▢▢▢▢ FITNESS

19 SATURDAY

MEALS

B _____

L _____

D _____

S

WATER ▢▢▢▢▢▢▢ FITNESS

20 SUNDAY

MEALS

B _____

L _____

D _____

S

WATER ▢▢▢▢▢▢▢ FITNESS

21 MONDAY

MEALS

B _____

L _____

D _____

S

WATER ▢▢▢▢▢▢▢ FITNESS

NOTES

WEEKLY To-Do's

15 Tuesday

....
....
....
....
....
....

HAPPINESS RATING: ☆☆☆☆☆

16 Wednesday

....
....
....
....
....
....

HAPPINESS RATING: ☆☆☆☆☆

17 Thursday

....
....
....
....
....
....

HAPPINESS RATING: ☆☆☆☆☆

18 Friday

....
....
....
....
....
....

HAPPINESS RATING: ☆☆☆☆☆

19 Saturday

....
....
....
....
....
....

HAPPINESS RATING: ☆☆☆☆☆

20 Sunday

....
....
....
....
....
....

HAPPINESS RATING: ☆☆☆☆☆

21 Monday

....
....
....

HAPPINESS RATING: ☆☆☆☆☆

WEEKLY *Food & Workout Tracker*

PLAN & TRACK YOUR MEALS & WORKOUTS

22 TUESDAY

MEALS

B _____
L _____
D _____
S

WATER ☐☐☐☐☐☐☐ FITNESS

23 WEDNESDAY

MEALS

B _____
L _____
D _____
S

WATER ☐☐☐☐☐☐☐ FITNESS

24 THURSDAY

MEALS

B _____
L _____
D _____
S

WATER ☐☐☐☐☐☐☐ FITNESS

25 FRIDAY

MEALS

B _____
L _____
D _____
S

WATER ☐☐☐☐☐☐☐ FITNESS

26 SATURDAY

MEALS

B _____
L _____
D _____
S

WATER ☐☐☐☐☐☐☐ FITNESS

27 SUNDAY

MEALS

B _____
L _____
D _____
S

WATER ☐☐☐☐☐☐☐ FITNESS

28 MONDAY

MEALS

B _____
L _____
D _____
S

WATER ☐☐☐☐☐☐☐ FITNESS

NOTES

WEEKLY *To-Do's*

22 Tuesday

....
....
....
....
....

HAPPINESS RATING: ☆☆☆☆☆

23 Wednesday

....
....
....
....
....

HAPPINESS RATING: ☆☆☆☆☆

24 Thursday

....
....
....
....
....

HAPPINESS RATING: ☆☆☆☆☆

25 Friday

....
....
....
....
....

HAPPINESS RATING: ☆☆☆☆☆

26 Saturday

....
....
....
....
....

HAPPINESS RATING: ☆☆☆☆☆

27 Sunday

....
....
....
....
....

HAPPINESS RATING: ☆☆☆☆☆

28 Monday

....
....
....

HAPPINESS RATING: ☆☆☆☆☆

WEEKLY *Food & Workout Tracker*

PLAN & TRACK YOUR MEALS & WORKOUTS

29 TUESDAY

MEALS

B _____

L _____

D _____

S

WATER

☐☐☐☐☐☐☐   **FITNESS**

30 WEDNESDAY

MEALS

B _____

L _____

D _____

S

WATER

☐☐☐☐☐☐☐   **FITNESS**

NOTES

WEEKLY *To-Do's*

29 Tuesday

....
....
....
....
....
....
....

HAPPINESS RATING: ☆☆☆☆☆

30 Wednesday

....
....
....
....
....
....
....

HAPPINESS RATING: ☆☆☆☆☆

Thoughts/notes about the month:

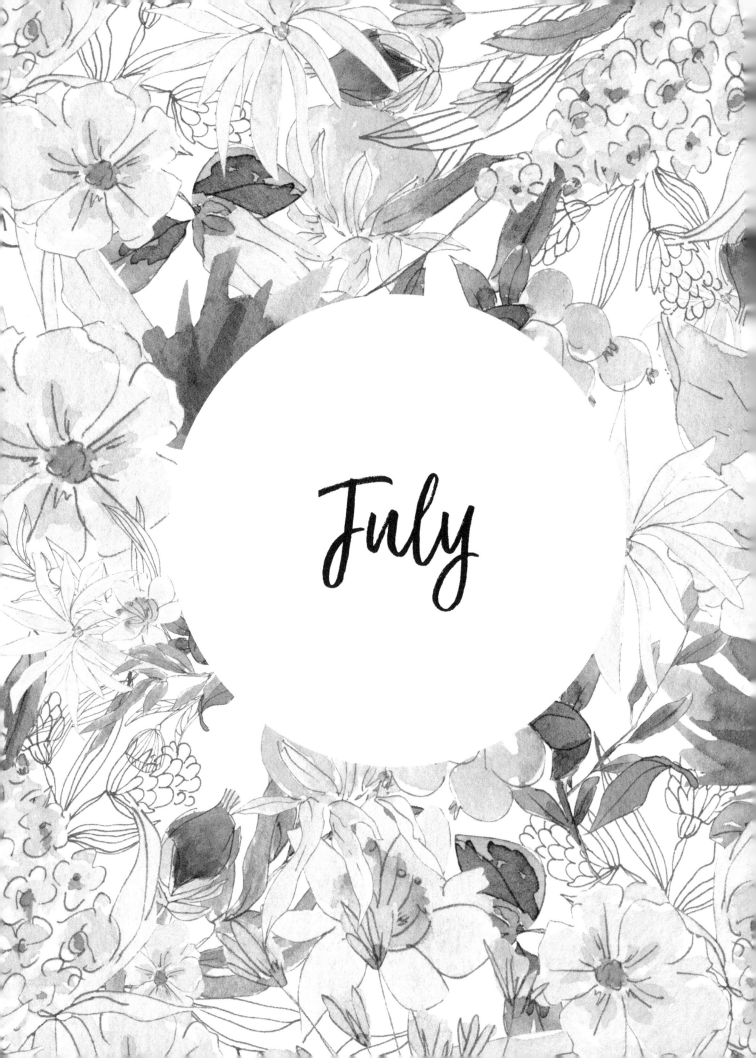

July

July

2021

Monthly Goals

Monthly Snapshot

Top Priorities

Tasks & Notes

July 2021

SUNDAY	MONDAY	TUESDAY	WEDNESDAY
4	5	6	7
11	12	13	14
18	19	20	21
25	26	27	28

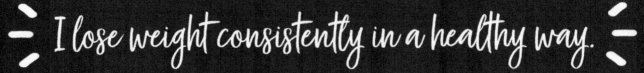

I lose weight consistently in a healthy way.

July 2021

THURSDAY	FRIDAY	SATURDAY	TO-DO LIST
1	2	3	○
			○
			○
			○
			○
8	9	10	○
			○
			○
			○
15	16	17	○
			○
			○
			○
			○
22	23	24	○
			○
			○
			○
			○
29	30	31	NOTES

July TRACKER

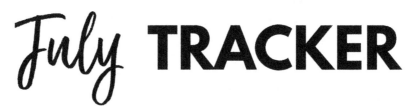

Use this tracker to document your measurements and weight loss progress.

WEIGHT:	MEASUREMENT	NOTES
ARMS		
CHEST		
WAIST		
HIPS		
THIGHS		
BICEPS		
SHOULDERS		

LBS LOST/GAINED:	INCHES LOST:	OTHER:

2 WINS LAST MONTH

WHAT TO DO BETTER/IMPROVE THIS MONTH:

1
2
3

3 THINGS I'VE LEARNED ABOUT MYSELF OVER THE LAST MONTH

Journaling / Notes / Brainstorming

WEEKLY *Food & Workout Tracker*

PLAN & TRACK YOUR MEALS & WORKOUTS

1 THURSDAY

MEALS

B _____

L _____

D _____

S _____

WATER ▢▢▢▢▢▢▢▢   FITNESS

2 FRIDAY

MEALS

B _____

L _____

D _____

S _____

WATER ▢▢▢▢▢▢▢▢   FITNESS

3 SATURDAY

MEALS

B _____

L _____

D _____

S _____

WATER ▢▢▢▢▢▢▢▢   FITNESS

4 SUNDAY

MEALS

B _____

L _____

D _____

S _____

WATER ▢▢▢▢▢▢▢▢   FITNESS

5 MONDAY

MEALS

B _____

L _____

D _____

S _____

WATER ▢▢▢▢▢▢▢▢   FITNESS

6 TUESDAY

MEALS

B _____

L _____

D _____

S _____

WATER ▢▢▢▢▢▢▢▢   FITNESS

7 WEDNESDAY

MEALS

B _____

L _____

D _____

S _____

WATER ▢▢▢▢▢▢▢▢   FITNESS

NOTES

WEEKLY *To-Do's*

1 **Thursday**

....
....
....
....
....

HAPPINESS
RATING: ☆☆☆☆☆

2 **Friday**

....
....
....
....
....

HAPPINESS
RATING: ☆☆☆☆☆

3 **Saturday**

....
....
....
....
....

HAPPINESS
RATING: ☆☆☆☆☆

4 **Sunday**

....
....
....
....
....

HAPPINESS
RATING: ☆☆☆☆☆

5 **Monday**

....
....
....
....
....

HAPPINESS
RATING: ☆☆☆☆☆

6 **Tuesday**

....
....
....
....
....

HAPPINESS
RATING: ☆☆☆☆☆

7 **Wednesday**

....
....
....

HAPPINESS
RATING: ☆☆☆☆☆

WEEKLY *Food & Workout Tracker*

PLAN & TRACK YOUR MEALS & WORKOUTS

8 THURSDAY

MEALS

B _____

L _____

D _____

S

WATER ▢▢▢▢▢▢▢▢   **FITNESS**

9 FRIDAY

MEALS

B _____

L _____

D _____

S

WATER ▢▢▢▢▢▢▢▢   **FITNESS**

10 SATURDAY

MEALS

B _____

L _____

D _____

S

WATER ▢▢▢▢▢▢▢▢   **FITNESS**

11 SUNDAY

MEALS

B _____

L _____

D _____

S

WATER ▢▢▢▢▢▢▢▢   **FITNESS**

12 MONDAY

MEALS

B _____

L _____

D _____

S

WATER ▢▢▢▢▢▢▢▢   **FITNESS**

13 TUESDAY

MEALS

B _____

L _____

D _____

S

WATER ▢▢▢▢▢▢▢▢   **FITNESS**

14 WEDNESDAY

MEALS

B _____

L _____

D _____

S

WATER ▢▢▢▢▢▢▢▢   **FITNESS**

NOTES

WEEKLY *To-Do's*

8 Thursday

....
....
....
....
....

HAPPINESS RATING: ☆☆☆☆☆

9 Friday

....
....
....
....
....

HAPPINESS RATING: ☆☆☆☆☆

10 Saturday

....
....
....
....
....

HAPPINESS RATING: ☆☆☆☆☆

11 Sunday

....
....
....
....
....

HAPPINESS RATING: ☆☆☆☆☆

12 Monday

....
....
....
....
....

HAPPINESS RATING: ☆☆☆☆☆

13 Tuesday

....
....
....
....
....

HAPPINESS RATING: ☆☆☆☆☆

14 Wednesday

....
....

HAPPINESS RATING: ☆☆☆☆☆

WEEKLY *Food & Workout Tracker*

PLAN & TRACK YOUR MEALS & WORKOUTS

15 THURSDAY

MEALS

B _____

L _____

D _____

S

WATER ▢▢▢▢▢▢▢   FITNESS

16 FRIDAY

MEALS

B _____

L _____

D _____

S

WATER ▢▢▢▢▢▢▢   FITNESS

17 SATURDAY

MEALS

B _____

L _____

D _____

S

WATER ▢▢▢▢▢▢▢   FITNESS

18 SUNDAY

MEALS

B _____

L _____

D _____

S

WATER ▢▢▢▢▢▢▢   FITNESS

19 MONDAY

MEALS

B _____

L _____

D _____

S

WATER ▢▢▢▢▢▢▢   FITNESS

20 TUESDAY

MEALS

B _____

L _____

D _____

S

WATER ▢▢▢▢▢▢▢   FITNESS

21 WEDNESDAY

MEALS

B _____

L _____

D _____

S

WATER ▢▢▢▢▢▢▢   FITNESS

NOTES

WEEKLY *To-Do's*

15 Thursday

HAPPINESS RATING: ☆☆☆☆☆

16 Friday

HAPPINESS RATING: ☆☆☆☆☆

17 Saturday

HAPPINESS RATING: ☆☆☆☆☆

18 Sunday

HAPPINESS RATING: ☆☆☆☆☆

19 Monday

HAPPINESS RATING: ☆☆☆☆☆

20 Tuesday

HAPPINESS RATING: ☆☆☆☆☆

21 Wednesday

HAPPINESS RATING: ☆☆☆☆☆

WEEKLY *Food & Workout Tracker*

PLAN & TRACK YOUR MEALS & WORKOUTS

22 THURSDAY

MEALS

B _____

L _____

D _____

S

WATER ☐☐☐☐☐☐☐☐   FITNESS

23 FRIDAY

MEALS

B _____

L _____

D _____

S

WATER ☐☐☐☐☐☐☐☐   FITNESS

24 SATURDAY

MEALS

B _____

L _____

D _____

S

WATER ☐☐☐☐☐☐☐☐   FITNESS

25 SUNDAY

MEALS

B _____

L _____

D _____

S

WATER ☐☐☐☐☐☐☐☐   FITNESS

26 MONDAY

MEALS

B _____

L _____

D _____

S

WATER ☐☐☐☐☐☐☐☐   FITNESS

27 TUESDAY

MEALS

B _____

L _____

D _____

S

WATER ☐☐☐☐☐☐☐☐   FITNESS

28 WEDNESDAY

MEALS

B _____

L _____

D _____

S

WATER ☐☐☐☐☐☐☐☐   FITNESS

NOTES

WEEKLY *To-Do's*

22 Thursday

....
....
....
....
....
....

HAPPINESS RATING: ☆☆☆☆☆

23 Friday

....
....
....
....
....
....

HAPPINESS RATING: ☆☆☆☆☆

24 Saturday

....
....
....
....
....
....

HAPPINESS RATING: ☆☆☆☆☆

25 Sunday

....
....
....
....
....

HAPPINESS RATING: ☆☆☆☆☆

26 Monday

....
....
....
....
....

HAPPINESS RATING: ☆☆☆☆☆

27 Tuesday

....
....
....
....
....

HAPPINESS RATING: ☆☆☆☆☆

28 Wednesday

....
....
....

HAPPINESS RATING: ☆☆☆☆☆

WEEKLY *Food & Workout Tracker*

PLAN & TRACK YOUR MEALS & WORKOUTS

29 THURSDAY

MEALS

B _____

L _____

D _____

S

WATER 🥛🥛🥛🥛🥛🥛🥛🥛 | FITNESS

30 FRIDAY

MEALS

B _____

L _____

D _____

S

WATER 🥛🥛🥛🥛🥛🥛🥛🥛 | FITNESS

31 SATURDAY

MEALS

B _____

L _____

D _____

S

WATER 🥛🥛🥛🥛🥛🥛🥛🥛 | FITNESS

NOTES

WEEKLY *To-Do's*

29 Thursday

....
....
....
....
....
....

HAPPINESS RATING: ☆☆☆☆☆

30 Friday

....
....
....
....
....
....

HAPPINESS RATING: ☆☆☆☆☆

31 Saturday

....
....
....
....
....
....

HAPPINESS RATING: ☆☆☆☆☆

Thoughts/notes about the month:

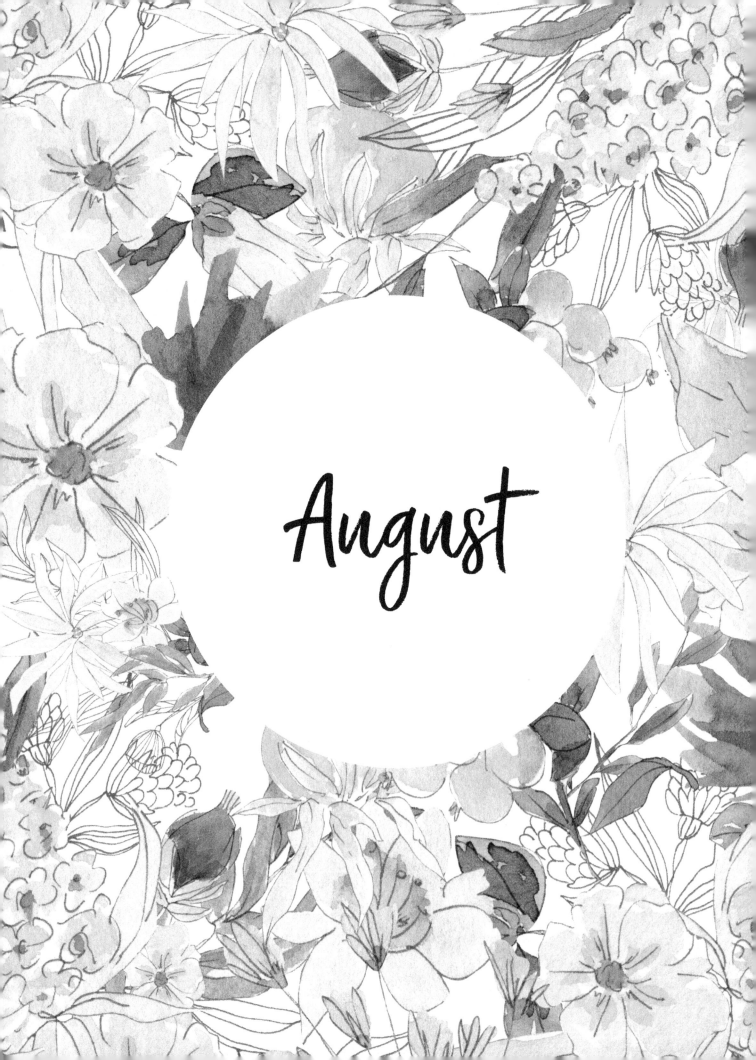

August

August

2021

Monthly Goals

Monthly Snapshot

Top Priorities

TASKS & NOTES

August

SUNDAY	MONDAY	TUESDAY	WEDNESDAY
1	2	3	4
8	9	10	11
15	16	17	18
22	23	24	25
29	30	31	

This situation is neither good nor bad. **IT SIMPLY IS.**

August

THURSDAY	FRIDAY	SATURDAY	TO-DO LIST
5	6	7	○
			○
			○
			○
			○
12	13	14	○
			○
			○
			○
19	20	21	○
			○
			○
			○
			○
26	27	28	○
			○
			○
			○
			○
			NOTES

August TRACKER

Use this tracker to document your measurements and weight loss progress.

WEIGHT:	MEASUREMENT	NOTES
ARMS		
CHEST		
WAIST		
HIPS		
THIGHS		
BICEPS		
SHOULDERS		

LBS LOST/GAINED:	INCHES LOST:	OTHER:

2 WINS LAST MONTH

WHAT TO DO BETTER/IMPROVE THIS MONTH:

1
2
3

3 THINGS I'VE LEARNED ABOUT MYSELF OVER THE LAST MONTH

WEEKLY *Food & Workout Tracker*

PLAN & TRACK YOUR MEALS & WORKOUTS

1 SUNDAY

MEALS

B _____

L _____

D _____

S

WATER ☐☐☐☐☐☐☐☐   FITNESS

2 MONDAY

MEALS

B _____

L _____

D _____

S

WATER ☐☐☐☐☐☐☐☐   FITNESS

3 TUESDAY

MEALS

B _____

L _____

D _____

S

WATER ☐☐☐☐☐☐☐☐   FITNESS

4 WEDNESDAY

MEALS

B _____

L _____

D _____

S

WATER ☐☐☐☐☐☐☐☐   FITNESS

5 THURSDAY

MEALS

B _____

L _____

D _____

S

WATER ☐☐☐☐☐☐☐☐   FITNESS

6 FRIDAY

MEALS

B _____

L _____

D _____

S

WATER ☐☐☐☐☐☐☐☐   FITNESS

7 SATURDAY

MEALS

B _____

L _____

D _____

S

WATER ☐☐☐☐☐☐☐☐   FITNESS

NOTES

WEEKLY *To-Do's*

1 Sunday

HAPPINESS
RATING: ☆☆☆☆☆

2 Monday

HAPPINESS
RATING: ☆☆☆☆☆

3 Tuesday

HAPPINESS
RATING: ☆☆☆☆☆

4 Wednesday

HAPPINESS
RATING: ☆☆☆☆☆

5 Thursday

HAPPINESS
RATING: ☆☆☆☆☆

6 Friday

HAPPINESS
RATING: ☆☆☆☆☆

7 Saturday

HAPPINESS
RATING: ☆☆☆☆☆

WEEKLY *Food & Workout Tracker*

PLAN & TRACK YOUR MEALS & WORKOUTS

8 SUNDAY

MEALS

B

L

D

S

WATER ☐☐☐☐☐☐☐ FITNESS

9 MONDAY

MEALS

B

L

D

S

WATER ☐☐☐☐☐☐☐ FITNESS

10 TUESDAY

MEALS

B

L

D

S

WATER ☐☐☐☐☐☐☐ FITNESS

11 WEDNESDAY

MEALS

B

L

D

S

WATER ☐☐☐☐☐☐☐ FITNESS

12 THURSDAY

MEALS

B

L

D

S

WATER ☐☐☐☐☐☐☐ FITNESS

13 FRIDAY

MEALS

B

L

D

S

WATER ☐☐☐☐☐☐☐ FITNESS

14 SATURDAY

MEALS

B

L

D

S

WATER ☐☐☐☐☐☐☐ FITNESS

NOTES

WEEKLY To-Do's

8 Sunday

....
....
....
....
....
....

HAPPINESS RATING: ☆☆☆☆☆

9 Monday

....
....
....
....
....
....

HAPPINESS RATING: ☆☆☆☆☆

10 Tuesday

....
....
....
....
....
....

HAPPINESS RATING: ☆☆☆☆☆

11 Wednesday

....
....
....
....
....
....

HAPPINESS RATING: ☆☆☆☆☆

12 Thursday

....
....
....
....
....
....

HAPPINESS RATING: ☆☆☆☆☆

13 Friday

....
....
....
....
....
....

HAPPINESS RATING: ☆☆☆☆☆

14 Saturday

....
....
....

HAPPINESS RATING: ☆☆☆☆☆

WEEKLY *Food & Workout Tracker*

PLAN & TRACK YOUR MEALS & WORKOUTS

15 SUNDAY

MEALS

B _____

L _____

D _____

S

WATER ⬚⬚⬚⬚⬚⬚⬚ FITNESS

16 MONDAY

MEALS

B _____

L _____

D _____

S

WATER ⬚⬚⬚⬚⬚⬚⬚ FITNESS

17 TUESDAY

MEALS

B _____

L _____

D _____

S

WATER ⬚⬚⬚⬚⬚⬚⬚ FITNESS

18 WEDNESDAY

MEALS

B _____

L _____

D _____

S

WATER ⬚⬚⬚⬚⬚⬚⬚ FITNESS

19 THURSDAY

MEALS

B _____

L _____

D _____

S

WATER ⬚⬚⬚⬚⬚⬚⬚ FITNESS

20 FRIDAY

MEALS

B _____

L _____

D _____

S

WATER ⬚⬚⬚⬚⬚⬚⬚ FITNESS

21 SATURDAY

MEALS

B _____

L _____

D _____

S

WATER ⬚⬚⬚⬚⬚⬚⬚ FITNESS

NOTES

WEEKLY *To-Do's*

15 Sunday

....
....
....
....
....

HAPPINESS RATING: ☆☆☆☆☆

16 Monday

....
....
....
....
....

HAPPINESS RATING: ☆☆☆☆☆

17 Tuesday

....
....
....
....
....

HAPPINESS RATING: ☆☆☆☆☆

18 Wednesday

....
....
....
....
....

HAPPINESS RATING: ☆☆☆☆☆

19 Thursday

....
....
....
....
....

HAPPINESS RATING: ☆☆☆☆☆

20 Friday

....
....
....
....
....

HAPPINESS RATING: ☆☆☆☆☆

21 Saturday

....
....
....

HAPPINESS RATING: ☆☆☆☆☆

WEEKLY *Food & Workout Tracker*

PLAN & TRACK YOUR MEALS & WORKOUTS

22 SUNDAY

MEALS

B

L

D

S

WATER ☐☐☐☐☐☐☐☐ FITNESS

23 MONDAY

MEALS

B

L

D

S

WATER ☐☐☐☐☐☐☐☐ FITNESS

24 TUESDAY

MEALS

B

L

D

S

WATER ☐☐☐☐☐☐☐☐ FITNESS

25 WEDNESDAY

MEALS

B

L

D

S

WATER ☐☐☐☐☐☐☐☐ FITNESS

26 THURSDAY

MEALS

B

L

D

S

WATER ☐☐☐☐☐☐☐☐ FITNESS

27 FRIDAY

MEALS

B

L

D

S

WATER ☐☐☐☐☐☐☐☐ FITNESS

28 SATURDAY

MEALS

B

L

D

S

WATER ☐☐☐☐☐☐☐☐ FITNESS

NOTES

WEEKLY *To-Do's*

22 Sunday

HAPPINESS
RATING: ☆☆☆☆☆

23 Monday

HAPPINESS
RATING: ☆☆☆☆☆

24 Tuesday

HAPPINESS
RATING: ☆☆☆☆☆

25 Wednesday

HAPPINESS
RATING: ☆☆☆☆☆

26 Thursday

HAPPINESS
RATING: ☆☆☆☆☆

27 Friday

HAPPINESS
RATING: ☆☆☆☆☆

28 Saturday

HAPPINESS
RATING: ☆☆☆☆☆

WEEKLY *Food & Workout Tracker*

PLAN & TRACK YOUR MEALS & WORKOUTS

29 SUNDAY

MEALS

B _____

L _____

D _____

S

WATER

FITNESS

30 MONDAY

MEALS

B _____

L _____

D _____

S

WATER

FITNESS

31 TUESDAY

MEALS

B _____

L _____

D _____

S

WATER

FITNESS

NOTES

WEEKLY To-Do's

29 Sunday

....
....
....
....
....
....

HAPPINESS
RATING: ☆ ☆ ☆ ☆ ☆

30 Monday

....
....
....
....
....
....

HAPPINESS
RATING: ☆ ☆ ☆ ☆ ☆

31 Tuesday

....
....
....
....
....
....

HAPPINESS
RATING: ☆ ☆ ☆ ☆ ☆

Thoughts/notes about the month:

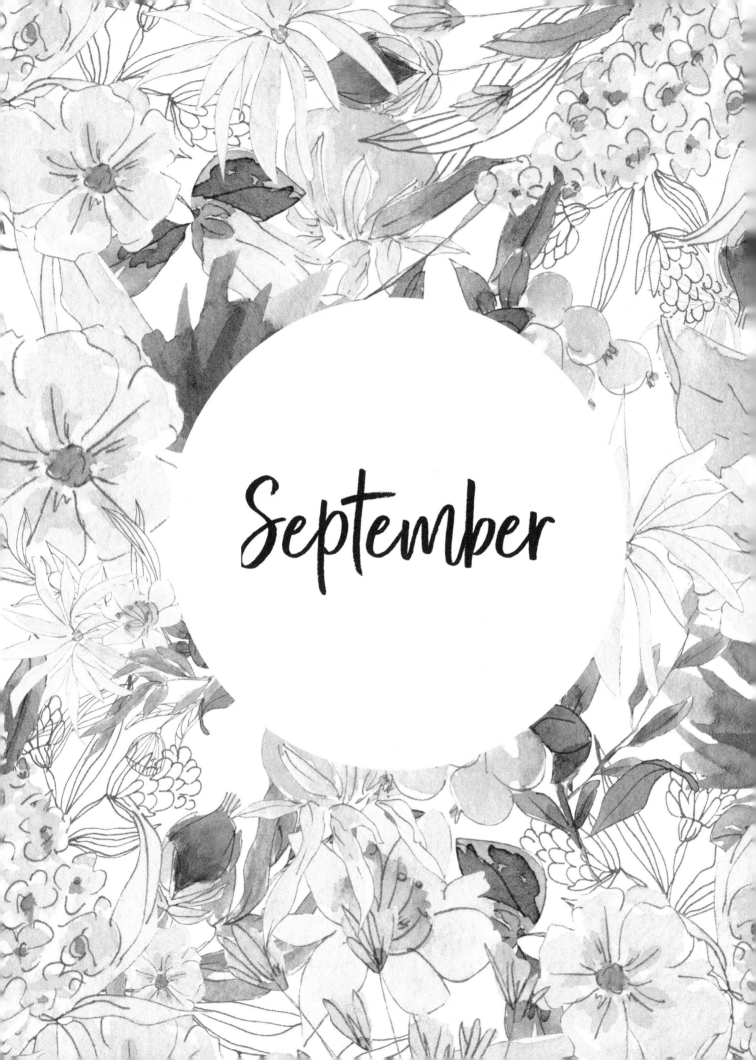

September

September

2021

MONTHLY SNAPSHOT

TOP PRIORITIES

TASKS & NOTES

September

2021

SUNDAY	MONDAY	TUESDAY	WEDNESDAY
			1
5	6	7	8
12	13	14	15
19	20	21	22
26	27	28	29

 I am SAFE inside my body.

September

THURSDAY	FRIDAY	SATURDAY	TO-DO LIST
2	3	4	○
			○
			○
			○
			○
9	10	11	○
			○
			○
			○
16	17	18	○
			○
			○
			○
			○
23	24	25	○
			○
			○
			○
			○
30			NOTES

September TRACKER

Use this tracker to document your measurements and weight loss progress.

WEIGHT:	MEASUREMENT	NOTES
ARMS		
CHEST		
WAIST		
HIPS		
THIGHS		
BICEPS		
SHOULDERS		

LBS LOST/GAINED:	INCHES LOST:	OTHER:

2 WINS LAST MONTH

WHAT TO DO BETTER/IMPROVE THIS MONTH:

1
2
3

3 THINGS I'VE LEARNED ABOUT MYSELF OVER THE LAST MONTH

Journaling / Notes / Brainstorming

WEEKLY *Food & Workout Tracker*

PLAN & TRACK YOUR MEALS & WORKOUTS

1 WEDNESDAY

MEALS

B _____

L _____

D _____

S

WATER ▢▢▢▢▢▢▢   FITNESS

2 THURSDAY

MEALS

B _____

L _____

D _____

S

WATER ▢▢▢▢▢▢▢   FITNESS

3 FRIDAY

MEALS

B _____

L _____

D _____

S

WATER ▢▢▢▢▢▢▢   FITNESS

4 SATURDAY

MEALS

B _____

L _____

D _____

S

WATER ▢▢▢▢▢▢▢   FITNESS

5 SUNDAY

MEALS

B _____

L _____

D _____

S

WATER ▢▢▢▢▢▢▢   FITNESS

6 MONDAY

MEALS

B _____

L _____

D _____

S

WATER ▢▢▢▢▢▢▢   FITNESS

7 TUESDAY

MEALS

B _____

L _____

D _____

S

WATER ▢▢▢▢▢▢▢   FITNESS

NOTES

WEEKLY To-Do's

1 Wednesday

....
....
....
....
....

HAPPINESS RATING: ☆ ☆ ☆ ☆ ☆

2 Thursday

....
....
....
....
....

HAPPINESS RATING: ☆ ☆ ☆ ☆ ☆

3 Friday

....
....
....
....
....

HAPPINESS RATING: ☆ ☆ ☆ ☆ ☆

4 Saturday

....
....
....
....
....

HAPPINESS RATING: ☆ ☆ ☆ ☆ ☆

5 Sunday

....
....
....
....
....

HAPPINESS RATING: ☆ ☆ ☆ ☆ ☆

6 Monday

....
....
....
....
....

HAPPINESS RATING: ☆ ☆ ☆ ☆ ☆

7 Tuesday

....
....
....

HAPPINESS RATING: ☆ ☆ ☆ ☆ ☆

WEEKLY *Food & Workout Tracker*

PLAN & TRACK YOUR MEALS & WORKOUTS

8 WEDNESDAY

MEALS

B _____
L _____
D _____
S _____

WATER ☐☐☐☐☐☐☐ FITNESS

9 THURSDAY

MEALS

B _____
L _____
D _____
S _____

WATER ☐☐☐☐☐☐☐ FITNESS

10 FRIDAY

MEALS

B _____
L _____
D _____
S _____

WATER ☐☐☐☐☐☐☐ FITNESS

11 SATURDAY

MEALS

B _____
L _____
D _____
S _____

WATER ☐☐☐☐☐☐☐ FITNESS

12 SUNDAY

MEALS

B _____
L _____
D _____
S _____

WATER ☐☐☐☐☐☐☐ FITNESS

13 MONDAY

MEALS

B _____
L _____
D _____
S _____

WATER ☐☐☐☐☐☐☐ FITNESS

14 TUESDAY

MEALS

B _____
L _____
D _____
S _____

WATER ☐☐☐☐☐☐☐ FITNESS

NOTES

WEEKLY *To-Do's*

8 Wednesday

....
....
....
....
....
....

HAPPINESS RATING: ☆☆☆☆☆

9 Thursday

....
....
....
....
....
....

HAPPINESS RATING: ☆☆☆☆☆

10 Friday

....
....
....
....
....
....

HAPPINESS RATING: ☆☆☆☆☆

11 Saturday

....
....
....
....
....
....

HAPPINESS RATING: ☆☆☆☆☆

12 Sunday

....
....
....
....
....
....

HAPPINESS RATING: ☆☆☆☆☆

13 Monday

....
....
....
....
....
....

HAPPINESS RATING: ☆☆☆☆☆

14 Tuesday

....
....
....

HAPPINESS RATING: ☆☆☆☆☆

WEEKLY *Food & Workout Tracker*

PLAN & TRACK YOUR MEALS & WORKOUTS

15 WEDNESDAY

MEALS

B _____

L _____

D _____

S _____

WATER ☐☐☐☐☐☐☐☐ FITNESS

16 THURSDAY

MEALS

B _____

L _____

D _____

S _____

WATER ☐☐☐☐☐☐☐☐ FITNESS

17 FRIDAY

MEALS

B _____

L _____

D _____

S _____

WATER ☐☐☐☐☐☐☐☐ FITNESS

18 SATURDAY

MEALS

B _____

L _____

D _____

S _____

WATER ☐☐☐☐☐☐☐☐ FITNESS

19 SUNDAY

MEALS

B _____

L _____

D _____

S _____

WATER ☐☐☐☐☐☐☐☐ FITNESS

20 MONDAY

MEALS

B _____

L _____

D _____

S _____

WATER ☐☐☐☐☐☐☐☐ FITNESS

21 TUESDAY

MEALS

B _____

L _____

D _____

S _____

WATER ☐☐☐☐☐☐☐☐ FITNESS

NOTES

WEEKLY *To-Do's*

15 Wednesday

HAPPINESS RATING: ☆☆☆☆☆

16 Thursday

HAPPINESS RATING: ☆☆☆☆☆

17 Friday

HAPPINESS RATING: ☆☆☆☆☆

18 Saturday

HAPPINESS RATING: ☆☆☆☆☆

19 Sunday

HAPPINESS RATING: ☆☆☆☆☆

20 Monday

HAPPINESS RATING: ☆☆☆☆☆

21 Tuesday

HAPPINESS RATING: ☆☆☆☆☆

WEEKLY *Food & Workout Tracker*

PLAN & TRACK YOUR MEALS & WORKOUTS

22 WEDNESDAY

MEALS

B _____

L _____

D _____

S

WATER ☐☐☐☐☐☐☐ FITNESS

23 THURSDAY

MEALS

B _____

L _____

D _____

S

WATER ☐☐☐☐☐☐☐ FITNESS

24 FRIDAY

MEALS

B _____

L _____

D _____

S

WATER ☐☐☐☐☐☐☐ FITNESS

25 SATURDAY

MEALS

B _____

L _____

D _____

S

WATER ☐☐☐☐☐☐☐ FITNESS

26 SUNDAY

MEALS

B _____

L _____

D _____

S

WATER ☐☐☐☐☐☐☐ FITNESS

27 MONDAY

MEALS

B _____

L _____

D _____

S

WATER ☐☐☐☐☐☐☐ FITNESS

28 TUESDAY

MEALS

B _____

L _____

D _____

S

WATER ☐☐☐☐☐☐☐ FITNESS

NOTES

WEEKLY *To-Do's*

22 Wednesday

....
....
....
....
....

HAPPINESS RATING: ☆☆☆☆☆

23 Thursday

....
....
....
....
....

HAPPINESS RATING: ☆☆☆☆☆

24 Friday

....
....
....
....
....

HAPPINESS RATING: ☆☆☆☆☆

25 Saturday

....
....
....
....
....

HAPPINESS RATING: ☆☆☆☆☆

26 Sunday

....
....
....
....
....

HAPPINESS RATING: ☆☆☆☆☆

27 Monday

....
....
....
....
....

HAPPINESS RATING: ☆☆☆☆☆

28 Tuesday

....
....

HAPPINESS RATING: ☆☆☆☆☆

WEEKLY *Food & Workout Tracker*

PLAN & TRACK YOUR MEALS & WORKOUTS

29 WEDNESDAY

MEALS

B _____

L _____

D _____

S

WATER □□□□□□□ **FITNESS**

30 THURSDAY

MEALS

B _____

L _____

D _____

S

WATER □□□□□□□ **FITNESS**

NOTES

WEEKLY *To-Do's*

29 Wednesday

....

....

....

....

....

....

....

HAPPINESS
RATING: ☆☆☆☆☆

30 Thursday

....

....

....

....

....

....

....

HAPPINESS
RATING: ☆☆☆☆☆

Thoughts/notes about the month:

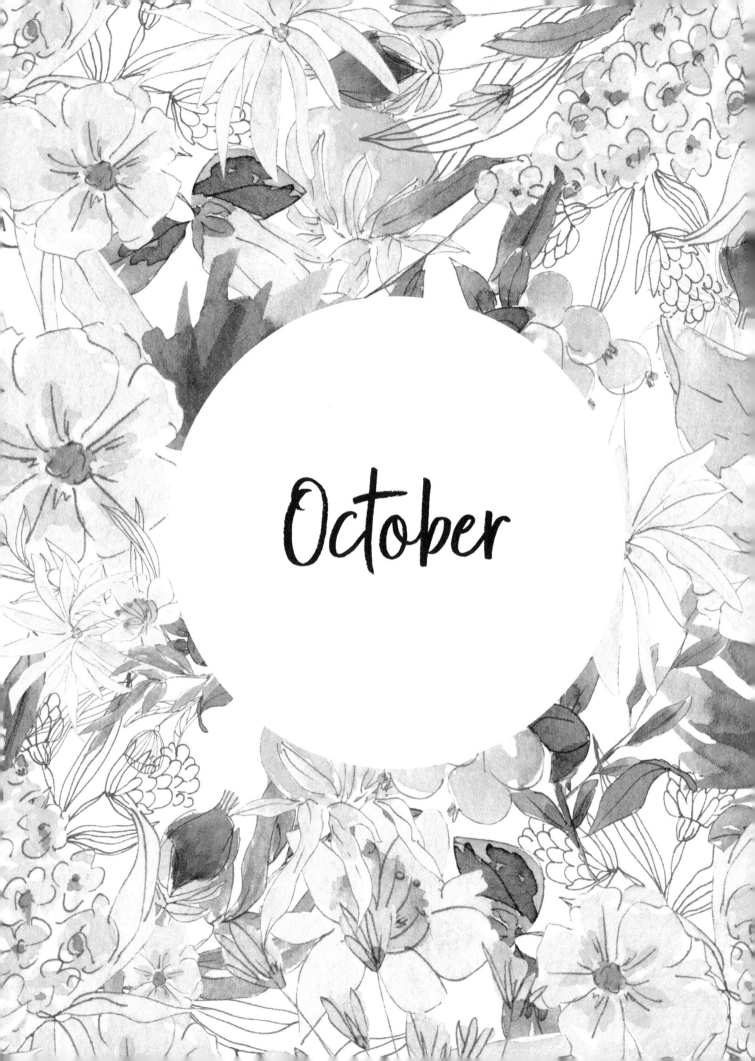

October

October

2021

Monthly Snapshot

Monthly Goals

Top Priorities

Tasks & Notes

October

SUNDAY	MONDAY	TUESDAY	WEDNESDAY
3	4	5	6
10	11	12	13
17	18	19	20
24	25	26	27

I EAT mindfully AND ENJOY EVERY BITE.

October 2021

THURSDAY	FRIDAY	SATURDAY	TO-DO LIST
	1	2	○
			○
			○
			○
			○
7	8	9	○
			○
			○
			○
14	15	16	○
			○
			○
			○
			○
21	22	23	○
			○
			○
			○
			○
28	29	30 / SUNDAY 31	NOTES

October TRACKER

Use this tracker to document your measurements and weight loss progress.

WEIGHT:	MEASUREMENT	NOTES
ARMS		
CHEST		
WAIST		
HIPS		
THIGHS		
BICEPS		
SHOULDERS		

LBS LOST/GAINED:	INCHES LOST:	OTHER:

2 WINS LAST MONTH

WHAT TO DO BETTER/IMPROVE THIS MONTH:

1	
2	
3	

3 THINGS I'VE LEARNED ABOUT MYSELF OVER THE LAST MONTH

Journaling / Notes / Brainstorming

WEEKLY *Food & Workout Tracker*

PLAN & TRACK YOUR MEALS & WORKOUTS

1 FRIDAY

MEALS

B _____
L _____
D _____
S _____

WATER ☐☐☐☐☐☐☐☐   FITNESS

2 SATURDAY

MEALS

B _____
L _____
D _____
S _____

WATER ☐☐☐☐☐☐☐☐   FITNESS

3 SUNDAY

MEALS

B _____
L _____
D _____
S _____

WATER ☐☐☐☐☐☐☐☐   FITNESS

4 MONDAY

MEALS

B _____
L _____
D _____
S _____

WATER ☐☐☐☐☐☐☐☐   FITNESS

5 TUESDAY

MEALS

B _____
L _____
D _____
S _____

WATER ☐☐☐☐☐☐☐☐   FITNESS

6 WEDNESDAY

MEALS

B _____
L _____
D _____
S _____

WATER ☐☐☐☐☐☐☐☐   FITNESS

7 THURSDAY

MEALS

B _____
L _____
D _____
S _____

WATER ☐☐☐☐☐☐☐☐   FITNESS

NOTES

WEEKLY *To-Do's*

1 Friday

HAPPINESS RATING: ☆☆☆☆☆

2 Saturday

HAPPINESS RATING: ☆☆☆☆☆

3 Sunday

HAPPINESS RATING: ☆☆☆☆☆

4 Monday

HAPPINESS RATING: ☆☆☆☆☆

5 Tuesday

HAPPINESS RATING: ☆☆☆☆☆

6 Wednesday

HAPPINESS RATING: ☆☆☆☆☆

7 Thursday

HAPPINESS RATING: ☆☆☆☆☆

WEEKLY *Food & Workout Tracker*

PLAN & TRACK YOUR MEALS & WORKOUTS

8 FRIDAY

MEALS

B _____

L _____

D _____

S _____

WATER ☐☐☐☐☐☐☐☐   FITNESS

9 SATURDAY

MEALS

B _____

L _____

D _____

S _____

WATER ☐☐☐☐☐☐☐☐   FITNESS

10 SUNDAY

MEALS

B _____

L _____

D _____

S _____

WATER ☐☐☐☐☐☐☐☐   FITNESS

11 MONDAY

MEALS

B _____

L _____

D _____

S _____

WATER ☐☐☐☐☐☐☐☐   FITNESS

12 TUESDAY

MEALS

B _____

L _____

D _____

S _____

WATER ☐☐☐☐☐☐☐☐   FITNESS

13 WEDNESDAY

MEALS

B _____

L _____

D _____

S _____

WATER ☐☐☐☐☐☐☐☐   FITNESS

14 THURSDAY

MEALS

B _____

L _____

D _____

S _____

WATER ☐☐☐☐☐☐☐☐   FITNESS

NOTES

WEEKLY *To-Do's*

8 Friday

....
....
....
....
....

HAPPINESS RATING: ☆☆☆☆☆

9 Saturday

....
....
....
....
....

HAPPINESS RATING: ☆☆☆☆☆

10 Sunday

....
....
....
....
....

HAPPINESS RATING: ☆☆☆☆☆

11 Monday

....
....
....
....
....

HAPPINESS RATING: ☆☆☆☆☆

12 Tuesday

....
....
....
....
....

HAPPINESS RATING: ☆☆☆☆☆

13 Wednesday

....
....
....
....
....

HAPPINESS RATING: ☆☆☆☆☆

14 Thursday

....
....
....

HAPPINESS RATING: ☆☆☆☆☆

WEEKLY *Food & Workout Tracker*

PLAN & TRACK YOUR MEALS & WORKOUTS

15 FRIDAY

MEALS

B _____

L _____

D _____

S _____

WATER ☐☐☐☐☐☐☐☐   **FITNESS**

16 SATURDAY

MEALS

B _____

L _____

D _____

S _____

WATER ☐☐☐☐☐☐☐☐   **FITNESS**

17 SUNDAY

MEALS

B _____

L _____

D _____

S _____

WATER ☐☐☐☐☐☐☐☐   **FITNESS**

18 MONDAY

MEALS

B _____

L _____

D _____

S _____

WATER ☐☐☐☐☐☐☐☐   **FITNESS**

19 TUESDAY

MEALS

B _____

L _____

D _____

S _____

WATER ☐☐☐☐☐☐☐☐   **FITNESS**

20 WEDNESDAY

MEALS

B _____

L _____

D _____

S _____

WATER ☐☐☐☐☐☐☐☐   **FITNESS**

21 THURSDAY

MEALS

B _____

L _____

D _____

S _____

WATER ☐☐☐☐☐☐☐☐   **FITNESS**

NOTES

WEEKLY *To-Do's*

15 Friday

HAPPINESS RATING: ☆☆☆☆☆

16 Saturday

HAPPINESS RATING: ☆☆☆☆☆

17 Sunday

HAPPINESS RATING: ☆☆☆☆☆

18 Monday

HAPPINESS RATING: ☆☆☆☆☆

19 Tuesday

HAPPINESS RATING: ☆☆☆☆☆

20 Wednesday

HAPPINESS RATING: ☆☆☆☆☆

21 Thursday

HAPPINESS RATING: ☆☆☆☆☆

WEEKLY *Food & Workout Tracker*

PLAN & TRACK YOUR MEALS & WORKOUTS

22 FRIDAY

MEALS

B _____

L _____

D _____

S _____

WATER ⬚⬚⬚⬚⬚⬚⬚⬚ FITNESS

23 SATURDAY

MEALS

B _____

L _____

D _____

S _____

WATER ⬚⬚⬚⬚⬚⬚⬚⬚ FITNESS

24 SUNDAY

MEALS

B _____

L _____

D _____

S _____

WATER ⬚⬚⬚⬚⬚⬚⬚⬚ FITNESS

25 MONDAY

MEALS

B _____

L _____

D _____

S _____

WATER ⬚⬚⬚⬚⬚⬚⬚⬚ FITNESS

26 TUESDAY

MEALS

B _____

L _____

D _____

S _____

WATER ⬚⬚⬚⬚⬚⬚⬚⬚ FITNESS

27 WEDNESDAY

MEALS

B _____

L _____

D _____

S _____

WATER ⬚⬚⬚⬚⬚⬚⬚⬚ FITNESS

28 THURSDAY

MEALS

B _____

L _____

D _____

S _____

WATER ⬚⬚⬚⬚⬚⬚⬚⬚ FITNESS

NOTES

WEEKLY *To-Do's*

22 Friday

....
....
....
....
....
....

HAPPINESS RATING: ☆☆☆☆☆

23 Saturday

....
....
....
....
....
....

HAPPINESS RATING: ☆☆☆☆☆

24 Sunday

....
....
....
....
....
....

HAPPINESS RATING: ☆☆☆☆☆

25 Monday

....
....
....
....
....
....

HAPPINESS RATING: ☆☆☆☆☆

26 Tuesday

....
....
....
....
....
....

HAPPINESS RATING: ☆☆☆☆☆

27 Wednesday

....
....
....
....
....
....

HAPPINESS RATING: ☆☆☆☆☆

28 Thursday

....
....
....

HAPPINESS RATING: ☆☆☆☆☆

WEEKLY *Food & Workout Tracker*

PLAN & TRACK YOUR MEALS & WORKOUTS

29 FRIDAY

MEALS

B _____

L _____

D _____

S

WATER 🥛🥛🥛🥛🥛🥛🥛🥛   FITNESS

30 SATURDAY

MEALS

B _____

L _____

D _____

S

WATER 🥛🥛🥛🥛🥛🥛🥛🥛   FITNESS

31 SUNDAY

MEALS

B _____

L _____

D _____

S

WATER 🥛🥛🥛🥛🥛🥛🥛🥛   FITNESS

NOTES

WEEKLY *To-Do's*

29 Friday

....
....
....
....
....
....

HAPPINESS
RATING: ☆ ☆ ☆ ☆ ☆

30 Saturday

....
....
....
....
....
....

HAPPINESS
RATING: ☆ ☆ ☆ ☆ ☆

31 Sunday

....
....
....
....
....
....

HAPPINESS
RATING: ☆ ☆ ☆ ☆ ☆

Thoughts/notes about the month:

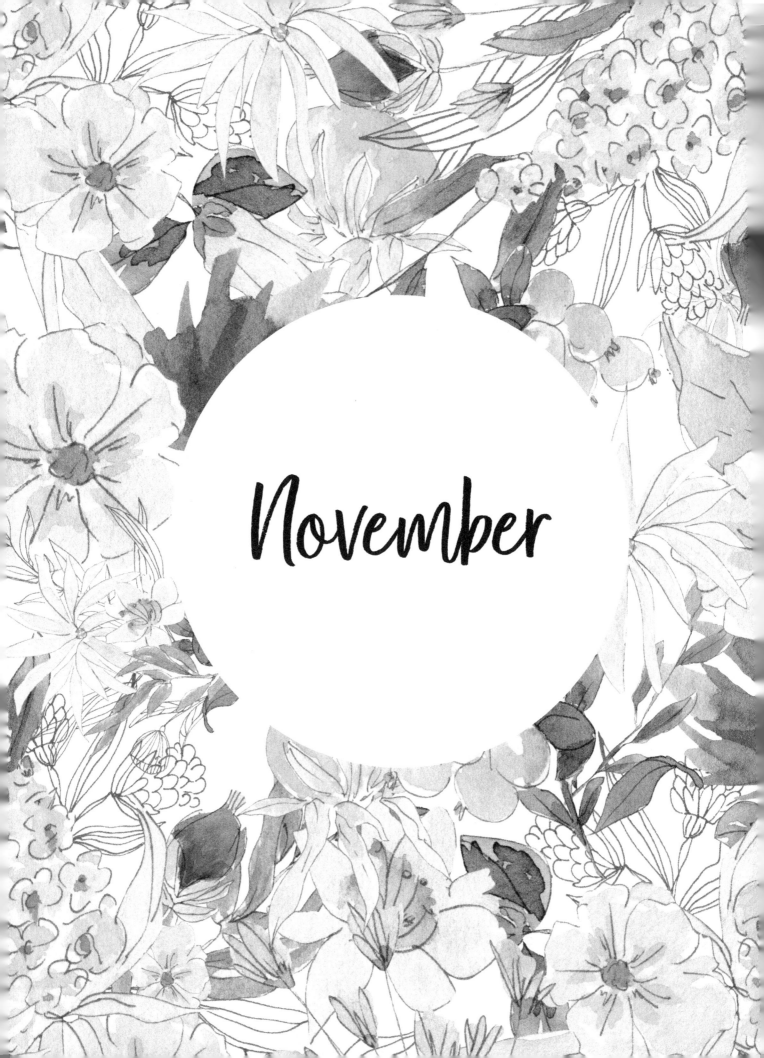

November

November

2021

MONTHLY SNAPSHOT

TOP PRIORITIES

TASKS & NOTES

November 2021

SUNDAY	MONDAY	TUESDAY	WEDNESDAY
	1	2	3
7	8	9	10
14	15	16	17
21	22	23	24
28	29	30	

All situations are TEMPORARY

November

THURSDAY	FRIDAY	SATURDAY	TO-DO LIST
4	5	6	○
			○
			○
			○
			○
11	12	13	○
			○
			○
			○
18	19	20	○
			○
			○
			○
			○
25	26	27	○
			○
			○
			○
			○
			NOTES

November TRACKER

Use this tracker to document your measurements and weight loss progress.

WEIGHT:	MEASUREMENT	NOTES
ARMS		
CHEST		
WAIST		
HIPS		
THIGHS		
BICEPS		
SHOULDERS		

LBS LOST/GAINED:	INCHES LOST:	OTHER:

2 WINS LAST MONTH

WHAT TO DO BETTER/IMPROVE THIS MONTH:

1	
2	
3	

3 THINGS I'VE LEARNED ABOUT MYSELF OVER THE LAST MONTH

Journaling / Notes / Brainstorming

WEEKLY *Food & Workout Tracker*

PLAN & TRACK YOUR MEALS & WORKOUTS

1 MONDAY

MEALS

B _____

L _____

D _____

S _____

WATER ☐☐☐☐☐☐☐   FITNESS

2 TUESDAY

MEALS

B _____

L _____

D _____

S _____

WATER ☐☐☐☐☐☐☐   FITNESS

3 WEDNESDAY

MEALS

B _____

L _____

D _____

S _____

WATER ☐☐☐☐☐☐☐   FITNESS

4 THURSDAY

MEALS

B _____

L _____

D _____

S _____

WATER ☐☐☐☐☐☐☐   FITNESS

5 FRIDAY

MEALS

B _____

L _____

D _____

S _____

WATER ☐☐☐☐☐☐☐   FITNESS

6 SATURDAY

MEALS

B _____

L _____

D _____

S _____

WATER ☐☐☐☐☐☐☐   FITNESS

7 SUNDAY

MEALS

B _____

L _____

D _____

S _____

WATER ☐☐☐☐☐☐☐   FITNESS

NOTES

WEEKLY To-Do's

1 Monday

....
....
....
....
....
....

HAPPINESS RATING: ☆ ☆ ☆ ☆ ☆

2 Tuesday

....
....
....
....
....
....

HAPPINESS RATING: ☆ ☆ ☆ ☆ ☆

3 Wednesday

....
....
....
....
....
....

HAPPINESS RATING: ☆ ☆ ☆ ☆ ☆

4 Thursday

....
....
....
....
....

HAPPINESS RATING: ☆ ☆ ☆ ☆ ☆

5 Friday

....
....
....
....
....

HAPPINESS RATING: ☆ ☆ ☆ ☆ ☆

6 Saturday

....
....
....
....
....

HAPPINESS RATING: ☆ ☆ ☆ ☆ ☆

7 Sunday

....
....
....

HAPPINESS RATING: ☆ ☆ ☆ ☆ ☆

WEEKLY *Food & Workout Tracker*

PLAN & TRACK YOUR MEALS & WORKOUTS

8 MONDAY

MEALS

B _____

L _____

D _____

S _____

WATER ☐☐☐☐☐☐☐☐   FITNESS

9 TUESDAY

MEALS

B _____

L _____

D _____

S _____

WATER ☐☐☐☐☐☐☐☐   FITNESS

10 WEDNESDAY

MEALS

B _____

L _____

D _____

S _____

WATER ☐☐☐☐☐☐☐☐   FITNESS

11 THURSDAY

MEALS

B _____

L _____

D _____

S _____

WATER ☐☐☐☐☐☐☐☐   FITNESS

12 FRIDAY

MEALS

B _____

L _____

D _____

S _____

WATER ☐☐☐☐☐☐☐☐   FITNESS

13 SATURDAY

MEALS

B _____

L _____

D _____

S _____

WATER ☐☐☐☐☐☐☐☐   FITNESS

14 SUNDAY

MEALS

B _____

L _____

D _____

S _____

WATER ☐☐☐☐☐☐☐☐   FITNESS

NOTES

WEEKLY To-Do's

8 Monday

HAPPINESS RATING: ☆☆☆☆☆

9 Tuesday

HAPPINESS RATING: ☆☆☆☆☆

10 Wednesday

HAPPINESS RATING: ☆☆☆☆☆

11 Thursday

HAPPINESS RATING: ☆☆☆☆☆

12 Friday

HAPPINESS RATING: ☆☆☆☆☆

13 Saturday

HAPPINESS RATING: ☆☆☆☆☆

14 Sunday

HAPPINESS RATING: ☆☆☆☆☆

WEEKLY *Food & Workout Tracker*

PLAN & TRACK YOUR MEALS & WORKOUTS

15 MONDAY

MEALS

B _____

L _____

D _____

S _____

WATER ☐☐☐☐☐☐☐   FITNESS

16 TUESDAY

MEALS

B _____

L _____

D _____

S _____

WATER ☐☐☐☐☐☐☐   FITNESS

17 WEDNESDAY

MEALS

B _____

L _____

D _____

S _____

WATER ☐☐☐☐☐☐☐   FITNESS

18 THURSDAY

MEALS

B _____

L _____

D _____

S _____

WATER ☐☐☐☐☐☐☐   FITNESS

19 FRIDAY

MEALS

B _____

L _____

D _____

S _____

WATER ☐☐☐☐☐☐☐   FITNESS

20 SATURDAY

MEALS

B _____

L _____

D _____

S _____

WATER ☐☐☐☐☐☐☐   FITNESS

21 SUNDAY

MEALS

B _____

L _____

D _____

S _____

WATER ☐☐☐☐☐☐☐   FITNESS

NOTES

WEEKLY *To-Do's*

15 Monday

....
....
....
....
....

HAPPINESS RATING: ☆ ☆ ☆ ☆ ☆

16 Tuesday

....
....
....
....
....

HAPPINESS RATING: ☆ ☆ ☆ ☆ ☆

17 Wednesday

....
....
....
....
....

HAPPINESS RATING: ☆ ☆ ☆ ☆ ☆

18 Thursday

....
....
....
....
....

HAPPINESS RATING: ☆ ☆ ☆ ☆ ☆

19 Friday

....
....
....
....
....

HAPPINESS RATING: ☆ ☆ ☆ ☆ ☆

20 Saturday

....
....
....
....
....

HAPPINESS RATING: ☆ ☆ ☆ ☆ ☆

21 Sunday

....
....
....

HAPPINESS RATING: ☆ ☆ ☆ ☆ ☆

WEEKLY *Food & Workout Tracker*

PLAN & TRACK YOUR MEALS & WORKOUTS

22 MONDAY
MEALS
B _____
L _____
D _____
S
WATER ☐☐☐☐☐☐☐ FITNESS

23 TUESDAY
MEALS
B _____
L _____
D _____
S
WATER ☐☐☐☐☐☐☐ FITNESS

24 WEDNESDAY
MEALS
B _____
L _____
D _____
S
WATER ☐☐☐☐☐☐☐ FITNESS

25 THURSDAY
MEALS
B _____
L _____
D _____
S
WATER ☐☐☐☐☐☐☐ FITNESS

26 FRIDAY
MEALS
B _____
L _____
D _____
S
WATER ☐☐☐☐☐☐☐ FITNESS

27 SATURDAY
MEALS
B _____
L _____
D _____
S
WATER ☐☐☐☐☐☐☐ FITNESS

28 SUNDAY
MEALS
B _____
L _____
D _____
S
WATER ☐☐☐☐☐☐☐ FITNESS

NOTES

WEEKLY To-Do's

22 Monday

HAPPINESS RATING: ☆☆☆☆☆

23 Tuesday

HAPPINESS RATING: ☆☆☆☆☆

24 Wednesday

HAPPINESS RATING: ☆☆☆☆☆

25 Thursday

HAPPINESS RATING: ☆☆☆☆☆

26 Friday

HAPPINESS RATING: ☆☆☆☆☆

27 Saturday

HAPPINESS RATING: ☆☆☆☆☆

28 Sunday

HAPPINESS RATING: ☆☆☆☆☆

WEEKLY *Food & Workout Tracker*

PLAN & TRACK YOUR MEALS & WORKOUTS

29 MONDAY

MEALS

B _____

L _____

D _____

S

WATER ☐☐☐☐☐☐☐   FITNESS

30 TUESDAY

MEALS

B _____

L _____

D _____

S

WATER ☐☐☐☐☐☐☐   FITNESS

NOTES

WEEKLY *To-Do's*

29 Monday

HAPPINESS RATING: ☆☆☆☆☆

30 Tuesday

HAPPINESS RATING: ☆☆☆☆☆

Thoughts/notes about the month:

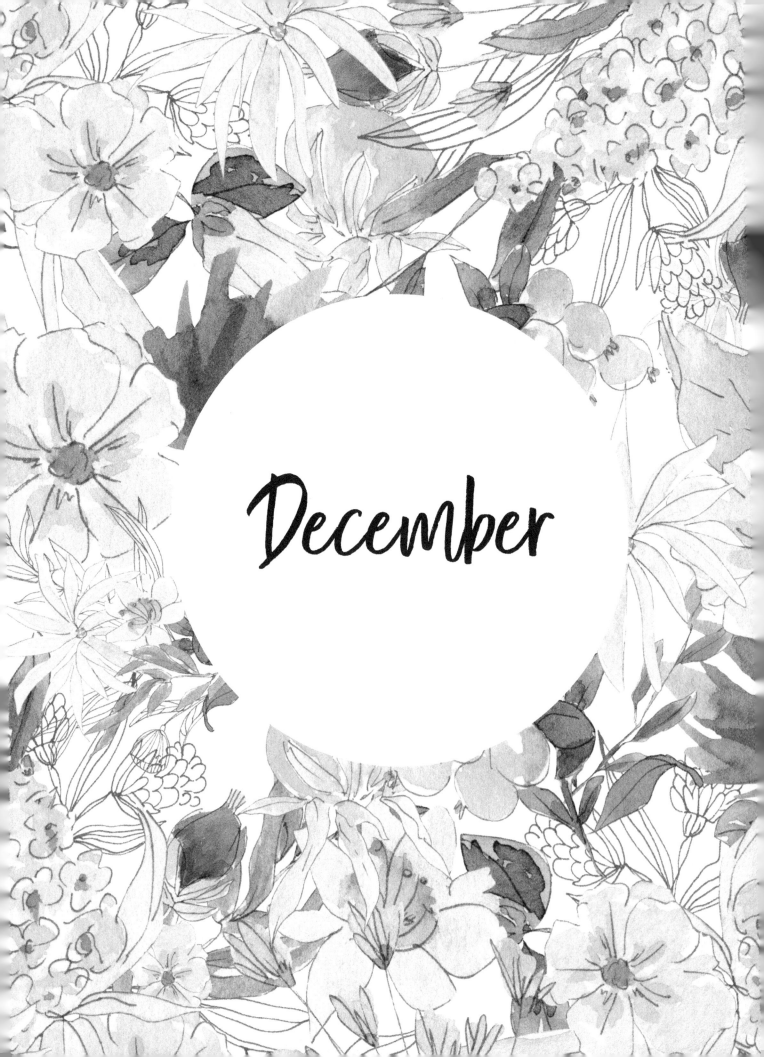

December

December

2021

MONTHLY SNAPSHOT

TOP PRIORITIES

TASKS & NOTES

December

SUNDAY	MONDAY	TUESDAY	WEDNESDAY
			1
5	6	7	8
12	13	14	15
19	20	21	22
26	27	28	29

TAKE 5 DEEP BREATHS *...and feel the energy return.*

December 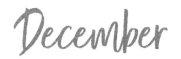 2021

THURSDAY	FRIDAY	SATURDAY	TO-DO LIST
2	3	4	○
			○
			○
			○
			○
9	10	11	○
			○
			○
			○
16	17	18	○
			○
			○
			○
			○
23	24	25	○
			○
			○
			○
			○
30	31		NOTES

December TRACKER

Use this tracker to document your measurements and weight loss progress.

WEIGHT:	MEASUREMENT	NOTES
ARMS		
CHEST		
WAIST		
HIPS		
THIGHS		
BICEPS		
SHOULDERS		

LBS LOST/GAINED:	INCHES LOST:	OTHER:

2 WINS LAST MONTH

WHAT TO DO BETTER/IMPROVE THIS MONTH:

1
2
3

3 THINGS I'VE LEARNED ABOUT MYSELF OVER THE LAST MONTH

Journaling / Notes / Brainstorming

WEEKLY *Food & Workout Tracker*

PLAN & TRACK YOUR MEALS & WORKOUTS

1 WEDNESDAY

MEALS

B _____

L _____

D _____

S _____

WATER ▢▢▢▢▢▢▢▢   FITNESS

2 THURSDAY

MEALS

B _____

L _____

D _____

S _____

WATER ▢▢▢▢▢▢▢▢   FITNESS

3 FRIDAY

MEALS

B _____

L _____

D _____

S _____

WATER ▢▢▢▢▢▢▢▢   FITNESS

4 SATURDAY

MEALS

B _____

L _____

D _____

S _____

WATER ▢▢▢▢▢▢▢▢   FITNESS

5 SUNDAY

MEALS

B _____

L _____

D _____

S _____

WATER ▢▢▢▢▢▢▢▢   FITNESS

6 MONDAY

MEALS

B _____

L _____

D _____

S _____

WATER ▢▢▢▢▢▢▢▢   FITNESS

7 TUESDAY

MEALS

B _____

L _____

D _____

S _____

WATER ▢▢▢▢▢▢▢▢   FITNESS

NOTES

WEEKLY *To-Do's*

1 **Wednesday**

....
....
....
....
....

HAPPINESS
RATING: ☆ ☆ ☆ ☆ ☆

2 **Thursday**

....
....
....
....
....

HAPPINESS
RATING: ☆ ☆ ☆ ☆ ☆

3 **Friday**

....
....
....
....
....

HAPPINESS
RATING: ☆ ☆ ☆ ☆ ☆

4 **Saturday**

....
....
....
....
....

HAPPINESS
RATING: ☆ ☆ ☆ ☆ ☆

5 **Sunday**

....
....
....
....
....

HAPPINESS
RATING: ☆ ☆ ☆ ☆ ☆

6 **Monday**

....
....
....
....
....

HAPPINESS
RATING: ☆ ☆ ☆ ☆ ☆

7 **Tuesday**

....
....
....

HAPPINESS
RATING: ☆ ☆ ☆ ☆ ☆

WEEKLY *Food & Workout Tracker*

PLAN & TRACK YOUR MEALS & WORKOUTS

8 WEDNESDAY

MEALS

B _____

L _____

D _____

S _____

WATER ☐☐☐☐☐☐☐   **FITNESS**

9 THURSDAY

MEALS

B _____

L _____

D _____

S _____

WATER ☐☐☐☐☐☐☐   **FITNESS**

10 FRIDAY

MEALS

B _____

L _____

D _____

S _____

WATER ☐☐☐☐☐☐☐   **FITNESS**

11 SATURDAY

MEALS

B _____

L _____

D _____

S _____

WATER ☐☐☐☐☐☐☐   **FITNESS**

12 SUNDAY

MEALS

B _____

L _____

D _____

S _____

WATER ☐☐☐☐☐☐☐   **FITNESS**

13 MONDAY

MEALS

B _____

L _____

D _____

S _____

WATER ☐☐☐☐☐☐☐   **FITNESS**

14 TUESDAY

MEALS

B _____

L _____

D _____

S _____

WATER ☐☐☐☐☐☐☐   **FITNESS**

NOTES

WEEKLY To-Do's

8 Wednesday

....
....
....
....
....

HAPPINESS RATING: ☆☆☆☆☆

9 Thursday

....
....
....
....
....

HAPPINESS RATING: ☆☆☆☆☆

10 Friday

....
....
....
....
....

HAPPINESS RATING: ☆☆☆☆☆

11 Saturday

....
....
....
....

HAPPINESS RATING: ☆☆☆☆☆

12 Sunday

....
....
....
....

HAPPINESS RATING: ☆☆☆☆☆

13 Monday

....
....
....
....

HAPPINESS RATING: ☆☆☆☆☆

14 Tuesday

....
....

HAPPINESS RATING: ☆☆☆☆☆

WEEKLY *Food & Workout Tracker*

PLAN & TRACK YOUR MEALS & WORKOUTS

15 WEDNESDAY

MEALS

B _____

L _____

D _____

S

WATER ☐☐☐☐☐☐☐☐   **FITNESS**

16 THURSDAY

MEALS

B _____

L _____

D _____

S

WATER ☐☐☐☐☐☐☐☐   **FITNESS**

17 FRIDAY

MEALS

B _____

L _____

D _____

S

WATER ☐☐☐☐☐☐☐☐   **FITNESS**

18 SATURDAY

MEALS

B _____

L _____

D _____

S

WATER ☐☐☐☐☐☐☐☐   **FITNESS**

19 SUNDAY

MEALS

B _____

L _____

D _____

S

WATER ☐☐☐☐☐☐☐☐   **FITNESS**

20 MONDAY

MEALS

B _____

L _____

D _____

S

WATER ☐☐☐☐☐☐☐☐   **FITNESS**

21 TUESDAY

MEALS

B _____

L _____

D _____

S

WATER ☐☐☐☐☐☐☐☐   **FITNESS**

NOTES

WEEKLY *To-Do's*

15 Wednesday

....
....
....
....
....
....

HAPPINESS
RATING: ☆☆☆☆☆

16 Thursday

....
....
....
....
....
....

HAPPINESS
RATING: ☆☆☆☆☆

17 Friday

....
....
....
....
....
....

HAPPINESS
RATING: ☆☆☆☆☆

18 Saturday

....
....
....
....
....
....

HAPPINESS
RATING: ☆☆☆☆☆

19 Sunday

....
....
....
....
....
....

HAPPINESS
RATING: ☆☆☆☆☆

20 Monday

....
....
....
....
....
....

HAPPINESS
RATING: ☆☆☆☆☆

21 Tuesday

....
....
....
....

HAPPINESS
RATING: ☆☆☆☆☆

WEEKLY *Food & Workout Tracker*

PLAN & TRACK YOUR MEALS & WORKOUTS

22 WEDNESDAY

MEALS

B _____

L _____

D _____

S

WATER ☐☐☐☐☐☐☐   FITNESS

23 THURSDAY

MEALS

B _____

L _____

D _____

S

WATER ☐☐☐☐☐☐☐   FITNESS

24 FRIDAY

MEALS

B _____

L _____

D _____

S

WATER ☐☐☐☐☐☐☐   FITNESS

25 SATURDAY

MEALS

B _____

L _____

D _____

S

WATER ☐☐☐☐☐☐☐   FITNESS

26 SUNDAY

MEALS

B _____

L _____

D _____

S

WATER ☐☐☐☐☐☐☐   FITNESS

27 MONDAY

MEALS

B _____

L _____

D _____

S

WATER ☐☐☐☐☐☐☐   FITNESS

28 TUESDAY

MEALS

B _____

L _____

D _____

S

WATER ☐☐☐☐☐☐☐   FITNESS

NOTES

WEEKLY To-Do's

22 Wednesday

....
....
....
....
....

HAPPINESS RATING: ☆☆☆☆☆

23 Thursday

....
....
....
....
....

HAPPINESS RATING: ☆☆☆☆☆

24 Friday

....
....
....
....
....

HAPPINESS RATING: ☆☆☆☆☆

25 Saturday

....
....
....
....
....

HAPPINESS RATING: ☆☆☆☆☆

26 Sunday

....
....
....
....
....

HAPPINESS RATING: ☆☆☆☆☆

27 Monday

....
....
....
....
....

HAPPINESS RATING: ☆☆☆☆☆

28 Tuesday

....
....
....

HAPPINESS RATING: ☆☆☆☆☆

WEEKLY *Food & Workout Tracker*

PLAN & TRACK YOUR MEALS & WORKOUTS

29 WEDNESDAY

MEALS

B _____

L _____

D _____

S

WATER ☐☐☐☐☐☐☐☐   FITNESS

30 THURSDAY

MEALS

B _____

L _____

D _____

S

WATER ☐☐☐☐☐☐☐☐   FITNESS

31 FRIDAY

MEALS

B _____

L _____

D _____

S

WATER ☐☐☐☐☐☐☐☐   FITNESS

NOTES

WEEKLY *To-Do's*

29 Wednesday

HAPPINESS
RATING: ☆☆☆☆☆

30 Thursday

HAPPINESS
RATING: ☆☆☆☆☆

31 Friday

HAPPINESS
RATING: ☆☆☆☆☆

Thoughts/notes about the month:

Made in the USA
Monee, IL
03 June 2021